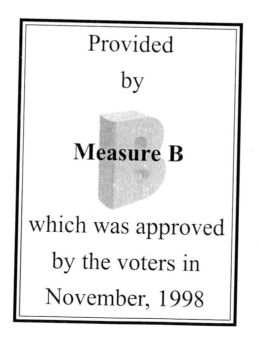

SHIATSU
FOUNDATION COURSE

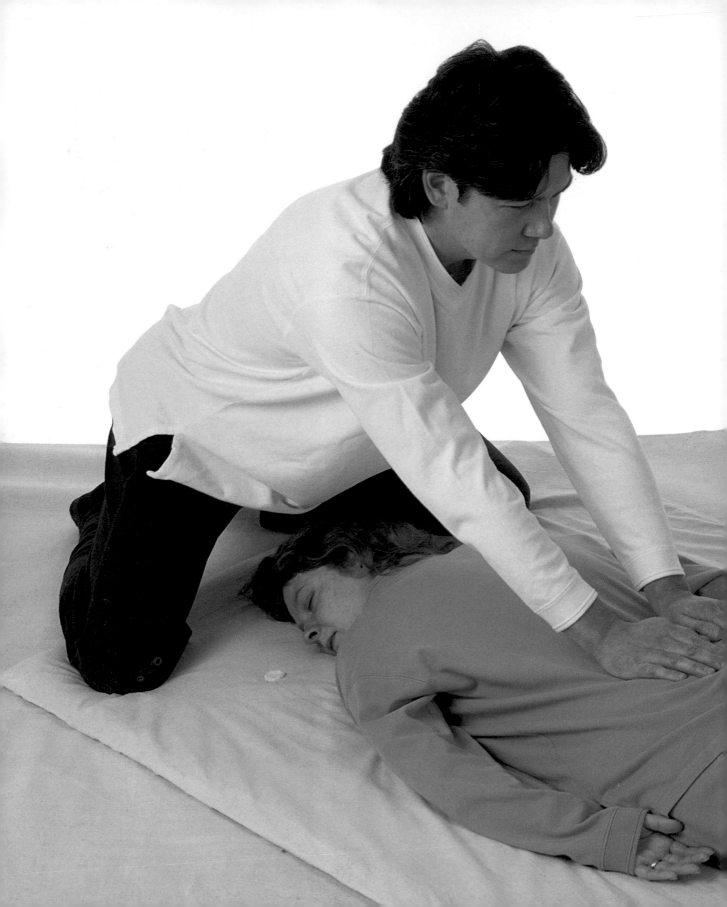

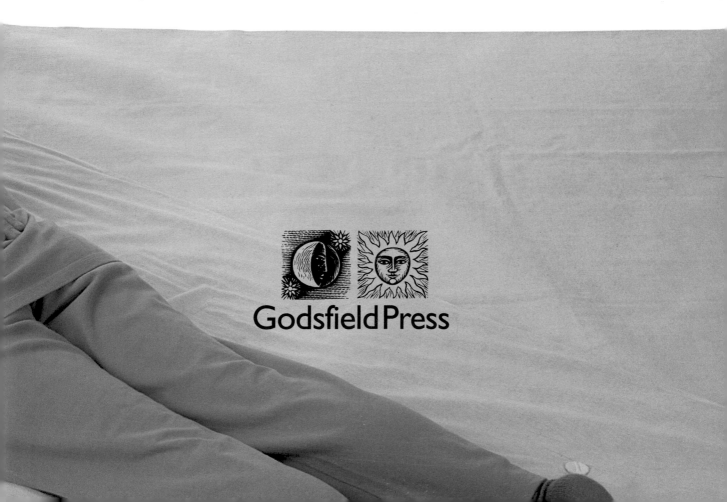

SHIATSU
FOUNDATION COURSE

CHRIS JARMEY

Godsfield Press

First published in Great Britain in 1999
by Godsfield Press Ltd, a division of
David & Charles Ltd, Laurel House, Station Approach,
Alresford, Hampshire, SO24 9JH, UK

10 9 8 7 6 5 4 3 2 1

Designed by Robin Whitecross
Photography by Alan Duns
Illustrations by Mei Lim

Printed in Italy by Lego SpA

ISBN 1899 434 194

The publishers would like to give a special thank you to Jane Pollard,
Jackie Monk, Patrick Davey, Jill Carter, Andrew Wilkinson and Max Jarmey.

Contents

Introduction

While few people in the West had heard of shiatsu before the mid-1980s, in the last 10 years it has experienced a rapid increase in popularity that outstrips the general growth of interest in complementary healing methods. Why this should be so is probably explained by the fact that many people are not only seeking alternative methods to combat disease and remain healthy – they are also looking for some sort of inner meaning and purpose to their lives.

So what is shiatsu, and how does it fulfil the dual role of a healing system and a method for personal development? Perhaps it is easier first to dismiss what it is not. It is not merely acupuncture without needles, or 'acupressure', although acupressure can be considered a subdivision of shiatsu. Neither is it simply an Oriental method of physiotherapy or soft tissue manipulation, although, if it is assessed purely on its range of physical techniques, it does incorporate aspects of these methods. The fundamental principle of shiatsu is that the giver, with clear mental focus, keeps in sustained stationary contact with a receiving person's body using thumbs, fingers, palms and sometimes elbows and knees, maintaining sufficient patience to wait for a response in the receiver's subtle energy or Ki (qi, ch'i) flow. A variety of stretching, rotating and levering techniques may be required to reduce the receiver's muscular and mental 'holding on', but essentially stationary pressure or 'connection' at the appropriate angle and depth is what differentiates shiatsu from massage.

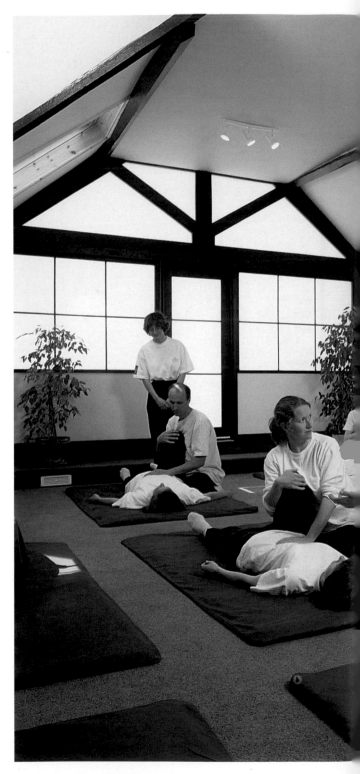

Shiatsu instruction in a class or from a personal tutor is the most effective way of learning this healing art.

The origins of shiatsu

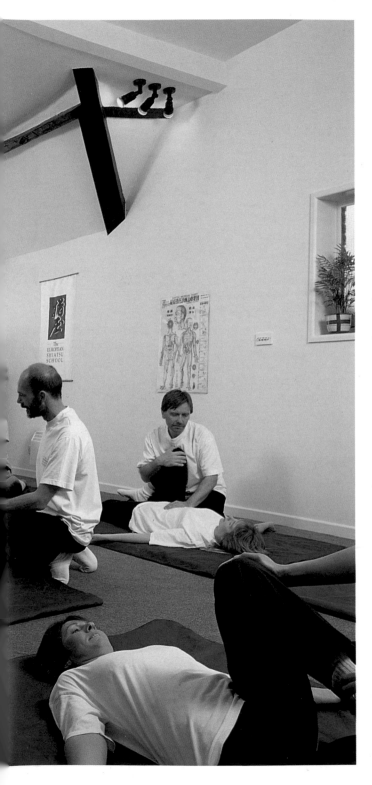

Shiatsu is a method of bodywork formulated in Japan in the 20th century as a development of various older forms of Chinese bodywork which are still practised in China and elsewhere today. In common with acupuncture and Chinese herbal medicine, these Chinese bodywork methods are all based on the principles of traditional Oriental medicine, which originated in ancient China. The degree to which shiatsu incorporates traditional Oriental medicine varies according to the style of shiatsu practised.

In the first half of the 20th century, Oriental medicine was generally discouraged throughout Japan in favour of Western medicine and many leading shiatsu exponents abandoned their heritage of Oriental medicine. However, some, along with many of their contemporaries in acupuncture, worked towards re-establishing Oriental medicine in Japan. Although the predominent style of shiatsu in Japan is still mostly based on Western medicine, the latter third of the 20th century has seen a complete reintegration of traditional Oriental medicine into many styles of shiatsu, particularly those now practised in the West.

Whichever style of shiatsu is practised, they all share many fundamental principles of how to apply pressure and stretch, and all have some techniques influenced by modern Western osteopathic or chiropractic methods, particularly in regard to lengthening muscles and mobilizing joints.

Today, shiatsu continues to grow and develop as its roots in Oriental medicine are explored ever more deeply. Modern practitioners and teachers are finding more methods of developing sensitivity to Ki and 'reading' the body, as well as innovative ways to apply effective technique based on the theories of Oriental medicine.

What is shiatsu about?

The quality and effectiveness of shiatsu depends upon the giver's state of mind. For example, shiatsu demands an ability to still and focus the mind in order to detect subtle changes within the receiver's vitality. Thereafter, it requires humility and skill to assist the natural healing process without superimposing the giver's expectations and judgements. It works more deeply if we understand that we cannot help restore true health effectively without acknowledging and responding to the receiver's own life energies. The shiatsu practitioner learns to listen to those energies and assist their natural inclination towards balance and harmony. Shiatsu is therefore about skilfully nurturing the body and mind's potential for revitalization.

The required level of mindfulness will naturally equip the giver with a greater ability to empathize with the receiver. This is because during the actual giving of shiatsu, the giver's mind is not in the future, predicting the outcome of the session, or in the past, trying to figure out what led the receiver to that point. The mind of the shiatsu therapist is trained to be in the here and now, which is the only time and space where we can hope to perceive reality. What the receiver is experiencing is happening only in the present, as the sum total of all preceding factors bringing them to this moment. Shiatsu brings both the giver and receiver to the same point in time – *now*. To be 'aware' *at* and *of* that point in time is the only condition in which empathy can be experienced.

We all feel empathy for another person at certain times, and this occurs when our consciousness rests for longer in the present. In shiatsu we aspire to keep our consciousness relating to the present for as much of the session as possible. Most methods of meditation and 'mindfulness' have the same purpose. In that sense, shiatsu is as much a practice for developing growth in awareness as it is a physical therapy. It is not mechanically physical, but rather physically mindful.

How to use this book

This book describes what is covered in a short shiatsu course for beginners and gives you an insight into how to develop the qualities of conscious touch required. It is not intended to bring you to the point of consummation of those abilities, for this requires a thorough in-depth training in shiatsu therapy lasting several years. Even then, such a course can only be expected to equip you with the theory, techniques and tools of shiatsu rather than the perfection of ability; only the sustained patient practice of shiatsu following a legitimate and thorough training will give you the necessary skill and humility to call yourself a professional shiatsu practitioner. However, for the relief of stress and minor ailments among family and friends via the inducement of a very deep level of relaxation, skills learned on a short foundation course can be applied immediately and to good effect.

What you learn during the early phases of any subject tends to become more ingrained than what is learned later on, and if you learn inaccuracies and poor form in the beginning it is consequently much more difficult to correct them later. The true purpose of this book is to supplement a good-quality foundation course which will set the novice student on the right track in the development of accurate and effective shiatsu technique.

You certainly cannot learn shiatsu solely from a book as detailed personal instruction and close supervision are necessary, but this book can function as a useful companion to a fully accredited foundation course or as an inspiration to embark upon such a course. It can then serve as a reminder of the basic shiatsu technique and principles, which will remain the same whatever level you take your shiatsu to. If in months or years to come you look back through this book and find that what you are doing under the name of shiatsu bears little relation to what is said within it, that is the time to reread it carefully. This is not to say that this book represents the last word on shiatsu technique, but it does elucidate the factors which make shiatsu what it is. Feel free to develop new techniques or reinterpret the theory as you gain experience; once you are truly skilled there are no limits to the possibilities of adding to shiatsu. Just be careful not to let go of the core. A solid snowball will grow as it rolls, but not if its original core melts.

Beyond the foundation course

Once you have completed a thorough shiatsu foundation course you may decide to study to full practitioner level in order to gain a deeper understanding of shiatsu practice and theory, along with a greater degree of sensitivity to Ki imbalances through the development of diagnostic skills. A practitioner course will teach you a wide range of practical techniques, including ways to affect all the Ki channels throughout the body, therapeutic stretching, how to develop your own style and treatments for a variety of health problems. You will also receive a thorough grounding in the theories of Oriental medicine and in Western anatomy, physiology and pathology as well as instruction on shiatsu diagnosis. Before receiving a diploma you will also carry out some form of supervised clinical work and learn how to manage a shiatsu practice.

While the curriculum for a diploma course may look very complex, the subject matter is actually very logical and builds naturally upon the foundation course curriculum. It is simple to master, provided you can give the necessary time to build up your touch sensitivity and read around the subject. The rewards are great, in that you will have a skill which will genuinely help others as well as yourself.

Contraindications to shiatsu

Because this is a book for beginners and meant only as a supplement to personal or class instruction from an experienced shiatsu teacher, you should only practise the techniques described in the following chapters on people who are fit and well. Do not practise on people who have problems such as osteoarthritis, rheumatoid arthritis, high or low blood pressure, contagious diseases, fever, cancer, heart disease, or any life-threatening conditions. You should also avoid parts of the receiver's body affected by varicose veins, burns, open sores, broken bones or bruises, tight or pulled muscles, ligament injuries or joint tenderness. Work around these areas instead.

In addition, do not give shiatsu to women during their first three months of pregnancy. Thereafter, for the remainder of the pregnancy you should avoid giving shiatsu below the knee. This is because there are several tsubos in this area which can initiate a miscarriage.

Your shiatsu mantra is: 'If in doubt, don't do it.' If you attend a proper series of shiatsu classes, you will learn when you can and cannot give shiatsu to people with particular problems. A book can never be a substitute for the one-to-one advice supplied by a personal teacher with whom you can discuss situations that arise.

HOW SHIATSU WORKS

While this foundation course book deals primarily with the practical aspects of effective shiatsu technique rather than with its theoretical basis, this chapter describes those key concepts of theory which will enable you to grasp why and how shiatsu works. It also considers the philosophical and medical principles of Yin-Yang theory and the theory of the Five Elements.

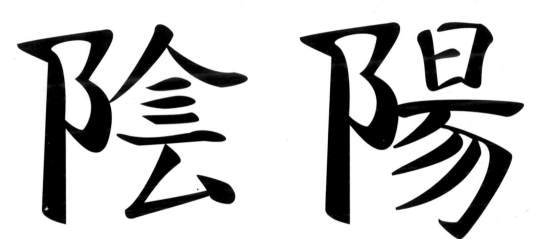

The characters for Yin and Yang

Yin-Yang theory

Oriental medicine is a complete reflection of traditional Oriental thinking and philosophy, all based on certain perceived universal truths such as the principles of Ki (Qi in Chinese) and Yin-Yang. In other words, in the Orient, medicine, art, politics, culture and philosophy are all based on a common understanding of the forces and cycles of nature.

Yin-Yang theory is an ancient Chinese conceptual framework for viewing and comprehending the world that was developed during the Yin and Chou dynasties, between 1500 and 221BC. The first textual reference to it is in the *Yi Jing* (or *I Ching*), the Book of Changes, around 800BC, and it is the aspect of change and of process which is at its heart. Yin-Yang theory is the foundation for understanding all phenomena, in particular health and disease. In Western philosophy contrary ideas oppose each other: if it is day then it cannot be night. However, in the Chinese model Yin and Yang oppose but also complement one another. Yin and Yang are contrary, but they can turn into one another and they each contain a small part of the other.

Putting the different components of the characters together, Yin is the cloudy or shady side of the hill and Yang the sunny side. On the Yang side it is light and warm and people are working, while on the shady side it is cold and dark and everyone is resting.

It is not, however, the case that Yin and Yang theory simply places phenomena into fixed categories; it is a way of explaining dynamic processes. Yin and Yang are relative terms, so, for example, a 100 watt light bulb is more Yang than a 30 watt bulb, but it is more Yin than the sun. To say that an apple, for instance, is Yin would be incorrect. It may be Yin (that is, colder) in relation to a steaming bowl of soup, or Yang (warmer) in relation to a tub of ice cream.

It doesn't make sense to talk of Yin except in relation to Yang; without the one the other is incomplete. In the Taiji symbol of Yin-Yang, Yang is the white part of the symbol and Yin the black. The two components coil around each other and interpenetrate; the white part of the symbol contains a black spot and the black part a white one. Nothing is ever entirely Yin or Yang but each contains something of the other, which may grow so that eventually each can become its opposite.

Yin and Yang symbol

Yin and Yang phenomena can themselves be further divided. For example, day is Yang compared to night, but a day may be divided into morning and afternoon. Morning, when the sun is rising, is more Yang than the afternoon, when the sun is setting, so morning is Yang and afternoon is Yin. Morning turns into afternoon, and in the same way Yang turns into Yin, and Yin into Yang. Day becomes night, summer turns to winter, our bodies move then rest, we are warm then

YIN AND YANG QUALITIES	
YIN	**YANG**
Darkness	Light
Cold	Heat
Rest	Movement
Moon	Sun
Earth	Heaven
West (sun sets)	East (sun rises)
North	South
Matter/substance	Energy/thought
Solid/liquid	Vapour/gas
Condensation	Evaporation
Contraction	Expansion
Descending	Rising
Below	Above
Form	Activity
Water	Fire
Yielding	Resistant
Soft	Hard
Passive	Aggressive
Introverted	Outgoing
Quiet	Loud
Slow	Fast
Wet	Dry
Chronic	Acute

cool, we wake and sleep. The movement from Yin to Yang is cyclical. The Chinese philosopher Chu Hsi wrote: 'The retreat of Yang IS the birth of Yin; it is not that once Yang has retreated a Yin separate from it is born . . . You can look at Yin-Yang as single or as twofold. Seen as twofold it divides into Yin and Yang; seen as single, it is simply a waxing and waning.' In the Taiji symbol, Yin is born where Yang reaches its peak, and vice versa.

Another way of looking at Yin and Yang is to regard them as different states or stages of being. In the course of the cyclical movement from Yang to Yin and back again, matter takes on different forms. For example, day turns to night and during the day the sun evaporates water from the earth and seas, forming vapour which condenses as evening approaches and is precipitated as dew during the cool of the night. That which evaporates, rises and is less substantial or formless is Yang in relation to that which condenses, falls downwards, is substantial and has form, which is Yin. To take this a little further, that which is non-material, more refined, less tangible, energetic rather than solid is Yang in relation to what is solid, material, grosser and tangible, which is Yin.

The interaction of Yin and Yang

There are four main ways in which Yin and Yang are related: they oppose one another; they complement one another; they can consume one another; they can transform into one another. In addition they are infinitely divisible.

Yin and Yang are opposites

As opposites, they struggle against one another and keep one another in check. Cold cools down heat: cooling drinks refresh on a hot day. Heat warms up cold: a fire heats you up on a cold day. This is the basis of treatment in Oriental medicine: if you have a hot condition, treatment should be cooling and vice versa. Treatment opposes one force with a contrary one.

The struggle between Yin and Yang results in a state of dynamic balance. In the body, as in other spheres, the balance is constantly changing. Take body temperature, for example: it is basically stable, but within a certain narrow range it fluctuates. If it fluctuates beyond that particular range, the physiological balance of the body is lost and disease arises.

The opposition of Yin and Yang within us powers our growth, development, maturation, ageing and decay. Relative balance within a restricted range brings about health and the loss of that balance brings about disease.

Yin and Yang are interdependent

As shown in the Taiji symbol, out of Yang comes Yin, out of Yin comes Yang. Each promotes the other, each brings the other into being. Without the one the other cannot exist.

Yin and Yang can consume one another

This means that where Yin predominates it will overwhelm and use up Yang and vice versa. For the body to work normally and keep itself warm (Yang), it has to burn up part of its substance (Yin). On the other hand, producing nutrient substances for the body (Yin) consumes a bit of energy (Yang). If either the Yin or Yang aspects of the body go beyond the normal range, the result is either an excess or a deficiency of them, resulting in disease.

Yin and Yang can transform into one another

The cycle of day and night and the yearly seasonal cycles are examples of this. To quote from an ancient Taoist text called *Plain Questions*: 'Extreme Yin will necessarily produce Yang, and extreme Yang will necessarily produce Yin.'

Yin-Yang as a guide to diagnosis and treatment

The root cause of any disease is an imbalance between Yin and Yang and the basic principle of Oriental medicine and of shiatsu is to adjust the balance. If we can understand the nature of the imbalance correctly we can take the right steps to correct it. On their own Yin and Yang are not sufficient to understand the precise nature of imbalances, but understanding Yin-Yang is the first step. For details of anatomy, physiology and pathology seen in the light of Yin and Yang, see Appendix II, page 121.

Five Element theory

From Yin-Yang theory it is clear that the ancient Chinese view of nature and the universe is one that focuses primarily on change and process. Five Element theory, or Five Phase theory, as it is also sometimes called, is another part of this view of change and movement. According to this concept, all phenomena are products of the movement of five elements: wood, fire, earth, metal and water. These elements are not the fundamental components of matter, but rather descriptions of certain qualities which pertain to particular phases of change.

Wood

Wood is characterized by growth and by upward and outward movement; it is associated with the springtime, with morning and with initiating action. Its energy ascends and disperses. It gives the ability to plan, control and be angry. It relates to the Liver and Gallbladder. A loud or clipped voice, a greenish complexion and a rancid odour may manifest with a Wood imbalance. People with a predominance of Wood are usually assertive, authoritative and well-organized, but may be irritable.

Fire

The qualities of fire are of heat and upward movement. It represents energy at its peak and is associated with summer and with noon. Fire gives us the capacity for warmth and love. It relates to the Heart and Small Intestine and the Heart Protector and Triple Heater. The Heart houses the mind, the seat of consciousness, the origin of all thought and emotion. A reddish complexion, a laughing or tremulous voice and a scorched odour may manifest with a Fire imbalance. A person with a predominance of Fire is often warm and sensitive but may also be excitable and emotionally changeable.

Earth

Earth is associated with the late summer harvest, with fertility, and with bringing phenomena into being. It is also linked with late afternoon and decreasing activity. It gives us the capacity for intellectual thought and concentration (called 'Yi'). It relates to the Spleen and Stomach and so to nourishment, which encompasses the taking in and digestion of food and information, both physically and intellectually. A yellowish tinge to the complexion, a singing quality to the voice and a slightly sickly-sweet odour may manifest with an Earth imbalance. People with a predominance of Earth are often good listeners, but may have a tendency to worry.

Metal

This element represents decline and is associated with autumn, evening and the balance between activity and rest. It represents purification, elimination and reform; it gives us the capacity to take in new experience and to eliminate the old. Its energy descends and disperses. It relates to the Lung and Large Intestine. The Lung houses the Corporeal soul (called 'Po'), which gives us animal vitality and the ability to live in the present. Grief and sadness relate to Metal. The skin is an extension of the Lung, so the Metal element is associated with the idea of boundary, of the border between ourselves and others. A whitish tinge to the face, a weeping quality to the voice and a rather musty odour of decay may manifest with a Metal imbalance. People with a predominance of Metal can be very optimistic but may easily feel melancholic.

Water

Water is decline at its maximum. It is associated with night, with winter, with latency, with yielding, with cold and with downward movement. Its energy floats or suspends. It is the initial impetus to grow after the dormancy of winter and gives us the will to live and the urge to procreate. It relates to the Kidney and the Bladder. Fear is the emotion associated with Water. A bluish or black tinge to the face, especially below the eyes, a groaning quality to the voice and a putrid odour may manifest with a Water imbalance. A person with a predominance of Water may be self-possessed and able, but may become timid or fearful if the Water element is unbalanced.

On the whole, people do not fall neatly into a single category but tend to combine qualities from a number of different Elements which may vary at different times in their lives. For the interaction of the Five Elements, see Appendix III, page 122.

The concept of Ki and Channels (Meridians)

Shiatsu works by helping to harmonize the energy and vitality of the body and mind. We know that when we eat we acquire energy, and if we eat healthily we expect to have more vitality. We also know that our quality of breathing is directly related to our energy levels. But what is it that animates us so that we are able to breathe and eat, move around and think? Something other than food and air exists within all living things, causing them to be 'alive'.

Western traditions view our 'life force' as an esoteric phenomenon, generally accepted by us as a gift from greater powers. As such, Westerners have not tried to understand it to the extent their Oriental counterparts have. The Oriental traditions see our 'aliveness' and therefore our energy and vitality as much more to do with our interaction with surrounding nature and the universe. Taoist philosophy, on which the bulk of Far Eastern medicine is based, is a way of describing and understanding how we and our environment function together. It is concerned with understanding how all things are ultimately striving to maintain balance and harmony and the observation that absolute balance and harmony cannot exist, due to constant opposing forces at work throughout nature.

Western thought has a rich fund of detailed information pertaining to how we are affected by cosmological cycles, astrology being the obvious example. However, it seems that it is the Oriental philosophies which most clearly map out how nature and our body/mind are animated and function. Here, we can simply say that the difference between that which is alive and that which is not alive is the presence or absence of 'aliveness'. This 'aliveness' is called Ki in Japanese, Qi or Ch'i in Chinese and Prana in Sanskrit (an ancient language of the Indian subcontinent). As this book is about shiatsu, we will call it Ki.

While we are alive, Ki permeates every part of our body, keeping every bodily function alive. Although cells are dying throughout our body, they are constantly being replaced. The replacement of cells declines as we grow older until not enough of the essential ones necessary for correct organic functioning are replaced. At that time we malfunction and die. The more Ki that reaches the cells the less prone to decay they will be, so that an abundant supply of Ki to a cell means a healthier cell. However, it is not simply a question of quantity, but also of movement; Ki flows smoothly and abundantly in a cycle within healthy vibrant creatures. Unhealthy creatures are not vibrant, because their Ki is not flowing smoothly.

In the latter case, it may be that Ki is not present in sufficient quantity to generate enough momentum to allow for a smooth flow, resulting in some areas being starved of vitality while others stagnate and accumulate waste products, rather like insufficient water failing to flush debris from a pipe. Alternatively, it may be that too much Ki is accumulating in a particular area or function of the body, causing stagnation or hyperactivity and irritation there.

Imbalances of Ki quantity and circulation have many causes, including emotional disturbance, shock, abnormal environmental factors such as excessive heat or cold, extreme assault from virulent organisms, poisons, poor diet, incorrect use of the body (creating postural/organ stress), accidents and so on. A professional shiatsu practitioner will strive to identify the cause and the exact effect of that cause upon the person seeking treatment and will then apply shiatsu to enhance Ki where it is needed, disperse and or calm the Ki in areas where it is blocked or irritated and make sure it circulates smoothly. Based on the understanding of what caused the imbalance, the practitioner will usually give advice as to how to avoid situations or factors which exacerbate the problem.

To understand the essence of shiatsu, you need to understand that Ki flows everywhere throughout the living body but aggregates into 'channels' of more concentrated Ki flow. Over the millenia, the Chinese mapped out these channels, or 'meridians', and through centuries of observation noticed what happens when a channel does not flow in the way it should. Consequently, they devised ways of restoring the correct 'attitude' of the channels and the Ki within them. Modern shiatsu is still based on these core principles.

These channels or meridians run like rivers all over the surface of the body and deep into its interior, directing Ki into and from all the internal organs. Where one channel begins and ends, it continues into another channel, so that there is a continuous circuit. Sometimes a channel will also connect with one or more other channels elsewhere along its course. From the main or primary channels, streams divide off at intervals, which themselves subdivide into more streams to supply Ki to all the bodily structures, such as muscles, fascia, bone and so on. The channel system is like a vast matrix supplying Ki to, and allowing intercommunication of Ki between, all areas and functions of the body (see Appendix III, page 122). This is not dissimilar to the ever-dividing and spreading profile of our nervous system and circulatory systems.

In shiatsu, as in the other branches of Oriental medicine, the internal organs are related to a wide range of functions of both the body and the mind. As such, if you affect the Ki channel of the receiver of shiatsu in some way, there will, at some level, be an effect upon their bodily functions, emotions and psychological disposition. This is the essence of a shiatsu session: to help the person's Ki re-establish strength and a more harmonious free-flowing state through the skilled application of physical contact to the body surface, thus bringing all aspects of the body/mind into greater harmony.

The tsubos

At specific locations along the Ki channels there are 'gateways' or 'cavities' where Ki can open to

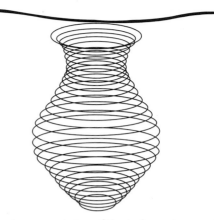

A representation of the tsubo vortex

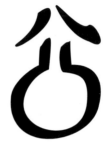

The Japanese character for tsubo

the surface. These gateways are known as 'tsubos' and are essentially pressure points where Ki can access the channel from outside the body, leave the channel to connect with the outside world or represent distortions in the channel flow, so that when 'activated' (by pressure, for example) the Ki can affect the channel and therefore some aspect of body/mind function.

A tsubo is a vortex of Ki which, if you could see it, would look like a vase-shaped swirl of energy with a mouth leading into a narrower neck which then widens into a broader belly. The Japanese written character for tsubo illustrates this concept perfectly (see above).

Each of the primary channels has a number of 'fixed' tsubos. Generations of documented observation have resulted in each being given a name, number and recognized action on the body and mind when stimulated. Some commonly used tsubos which can boost vitality and relieve minor ailments are listed in Appendix IV (page 125).

In addition to the fixed tsubos, there are 'transient tsubos' which come and go along the channels between the fixed tsubos. They arise where and when they do because there is either a lack of Ki or an excessive build up of Ki at that location and that point in time along the channel. Where the Ki is lacking, the tsubo will feel lifeless and 'empty', lacking vitality and elasticity. It may be stiff and lifeless or flaccid and lifeless. Sometimes it may be flaccid and lifeless on the surface and stiff and lifeless deeper down. Where the Ki is blocked and consequently overcrowded, there will be a feeling of fullness, tightness and constriction at that location, often accompanied by pain when touched there. Sometimes the full areas will feel warm whereas the deficient areas will feel cold.

Very occasionally, the shiatsu practitioner will feel active resistance on contacting a tsubo, even if the tsubo is deficient in Ki, thus making it difficult to discern whether it is full or empty. This is because surrounding Ki will rush to protect the empty, 'vulnerable' tsubo. This only happens when the tsubo is approached too quickly or too forcefully, which should not happen if your shiatsu is applied correctly.

Ki balance

To be alive is to have sufficient Ki to enable our body/mind to 'react' in some way; to be dead is to have insufficient Ki to react at all. The way Ki manifests in our actions and reactions depends upon what external factors are bearing down on us, what our immediate needs are and how emotionally and physically at ease we are within ourselves. So, if we possess sufficient Ki and are completely satisfied, our Ki will be evenly distributed throughout our body, smoothly transported through our network of Ki channels, giving us the appearance of being at rest. On the other hand, as soon as a need arises, such as hunger, we are no longer in a state of complete satisfaction. Hunger means we want food. As such, our Ki will aggregate into specific areas and functions of our body/mind (and therefore into specific Ki channels and tsubos) to enable us to get food. If the food is

just an arm's length away, very little Ki will need to be redistributed for us to eat. However, if we have to catch, kill, prepare, guard and eat our food, a lot more Ki will need to be reorganized within us. Once the hunger has been satisfied, our Ki distribution can return to its balanced state.

From this analogy, we can see that any activity we engage in results from a desire or need to fulfil ourselves. Getting food is an obvious example, but even the activity of drawing a picture results from a desire to draw it. That desire would not exist if we were totally fulfilled and satiated. We might draw the picture just to relieve boredom or because we have a powerful urge to create it, but whatever the specific motivation may be, the underlying thought is that we believe the picture should come into existence. Until the picture is completed to our satisfaction, we will invest a great deal of Ki into the functions which enable us to draw it. Once it is drawn, our Ki will return to balance.

So, all activity and therefore all movement of Ki within a living being results from need, and the fluctuation from need to fulfilment continues as long as life continues. It is perfectly normal and it explains why Ki moves more into certain channels and tsubos at any given time. As long as the Ki *does* return to normal, we remain healthy. However, if it remains stuck and does not rebalance itself, the seeds of ill health are sown. It can remain stuck because our intellect and our relationship to our environment is so complex that we do not necessarily know clearly what our needs are, nor when they are fulfilled. For example, do you eat only when you are hungry? Or do you sometimes eat in an attempt to satisfy a desire which you cannot even identify? Do you exhaust yourself trying to accumulate more food or money than you need, and if so, why is this?

The answers to such questions may be found through reflection, philosophy and psychology. What concerns the shiatsu practitioner is the effect this has on the distribution of Ki within the receiver's body and what he or she can do to help rebalance the Ki.

The Kyo-Jitsu principle

In shiatsu terminology, fullness or excess of Ki causing blockage or hyperactivity in a channel or tsubo is referred to as 'jitsu', whereas deficiency or emptiness of Ki resulting in hypoactivity or relative 'lifelessness' in a channel is known as 'kyo'. To further understand kyo, consider that every part of a living body seeks to be nourished by Ki and blood, so if insufficient Ki reaches any part, that part exhibits a 'need' for more Ki. Furthermore, a need (kyo) will eventually create a reaction (jitsu) somewhere, in an attempt to compensate for or meet that need. Kyo is therefore the underlying cause for jitsu. To reiterate the analogy of hunger, if the food supply is ample, there is no need to rush around urgently to fill the food cabinets. However, if the food runs out and we start to go hungry, we begin to focus a lot of energy and resources into procuring more food (the 'needy' kyo channel area is causing heightened activity or 'jitsu' elsewhere). When some family members start to grow dangerously weak from hunger, those who are able will go to extreme lengths to get food (greater kyo leads to more intense jitsu elsewhere). In a way, we are like a huge matrix that needs to be evenly spread, so when an imbalance in one area causes distortion in other areas a lot of energy is used in an attempt to restore equilibrium.

The Ki matrix of the body/mind, which is made up of our Ki channels, instinctively strives for balance; it wants smooth flow of Ki and a trouble-free existence. Our minds, our activities and our environmental influences sometimes work against that, yet our Ki matrix still strives for harmony within itself. It actually takes a lot of effort or adverse circumstance to overcome the harmony of the body. However, when the balance is lost, we become ill. The illness itself is an attempt to restore harmony, but sometimes the body/mind just does not have the final resources or resolve to get well without some outside help. Hence, we

have healing systems of various sorts, including shiatsu, which helps restore health or prevent ill health by keeping the Ki flowing smoothly throughout the channels, using techniques to meet the needs of the kyo and, if necessary, disperse or calm down the jitsu. In shiatsu, the words kyo and jitsu are usually restricted to describing the state of the channels and tsubos and are not used to describe anomalies in the organ functions, which are usually described as Yin-Yang imbalances, even though both channel distortions and functional imbalances sometimes amount to the same symptom.

So, any given channel will exhibit some areas that are more kyo and others that are more jitsu. In addition, you can expect any channel when viewed overall to err towards more kyo or more jitsu in relation to other channels. The whole 'matrix' is constantly fluctuating. A shiatsu therapist will find the most kyo channel and the most jitsu channel and focus their work on these two. By moving some of the Ki from the jitsu channel to the kyo channel, they will enhance the Ki within the kyo channel, therefore fulfilling its need for Ki.

The jitsu areas are more easy to find because they feel 'active' and react locally to pressure. Jitsu areas sometimes protrude from the surface. Kyo areas are more difficult to locate because they exhibit little or no reaction to touch and do not generally manifest an obvious presence on the surface, although the trained eye and touch can often see or feel kyo as a depression or 'sinking' into the surface. However, that is still more difficult than seeing that which protrudes or feeling that which reacts.

It is possible to develop a strongly jitsu state within one or more channels without there being an obvious underlying weakness or kyo. For example, certain external factors such as a cold wind blowing down your neck might cause the Ki in some of the channels running through that area to block or react in some way. This reaction is a response to the external influence, namely the wind, rather than some kyo elsewhere in the body.

SOME COMPARISONS OF KYO AND JITSU

Kyo	Jitsu
A 'need' which requires the Ki to be supported and strengthened	A bodily reaction representing its natural attempt to restore harmonious Ki flow
Underlying cause	Manifests as symptoms
Empty – requires filling	Full – requires emptying/dispersing
'Stagnation' in the channel due to the lack of Ki, being unable to sustain enough momentum for Ki circulation	'Stagnation' in the channel due to too much Ki occupying a confined area
Underactive, leading to flaccidity or stiffness	Hyperactive, leading to congestion, blockage and impenetrability
Below surface	Protruding from surface
Less obvious	More obvious
Slower to respond	Immediate response
Requires deep, sustained connection	Requires moving/active technique or to be left alone
Its tonification affects the whole person	Its dispersal affects localized body areas

However, if out of three people exposed to the same situation only one gets a stiff neck from Ki blockage, what is it about that person which is different from the other two? The answer is that that person had some underlying weakness compared to the other two people, which meant his resistance to wind was lower. So ultimately, if not immediately, jitsu always manifests out of a response to kyo.

Balancing kyo and jitsu distortions in the channels and tsubos constitutes the bulk of shiatsu technique application, although there are other facets to its practice. At foundation course level there is no need for you to worry too much about developing highly skilled methods to recognize and deal with kyo and jitsu; you can begin by simply recognizing where your touch is not welcome and avoiding those areas, while applying sustained contact to those 'appreciative' areas where you are able to tell that your touch is wanted. You can ask the receiver to tell you whether they want you to continue adding pressure to an area or whether they want you to move away from it – the jitsu areas will hurt them if pressure is applied. After some practice, you will begin to recognize the signs well before they have to tell you and thus your sensitivity will grow.

The effect of shiatsu on the autonomic nervous system (ANS)

Japanese character for human

Taken in its entirety, shiatsu therapy draws upon an extensive theoretical base and a range of practical approaches, and can offer an almost endless selection of techniques. However, a correctly applied shiatsu session consisting only of basic techniques will still have a tremendously positive effect upon the receiver, even without working specifically on the channels and without using the tools of diagnosis and the theory of Oriental medicine. It is this level of basic shiatsu application that this book sets out to describe. In a nutshell, shiatsu at any level is incredibly relaxing and revitalizing and it also strengthens the immune system. This is because it invokes the para-sympathetic response of the autonomic nervous system, which in simple terms means a deep relaxation response.

For our purposes here, there is no need for an exhaustive discussion of the physiology of the autonomic nervous system; it is sufficient to understand that we have physiological and psychological responses to threat which are more or less opposite to our reaction to safe and supportive situations.

When we perceive ourselves to be under threat, we become very alert so that we can rapidly assess the gravity and detail of the situation, thereby giving ourselves the optimum chance to counteract or escape from that which threatens us. Depending on the level of threat, we may be required to defend ourselves either by fighting it out or by running away. Under threat, our bodies will automatically send more adrenalin into the blood and more blood to the muscles, ensuring their optimum performance. Our breathing rhythm will accelerate to ensure enough oxygen gets to our muscles and brain, and our senses of hearing, seeing and smelling will become more acute. We become ready for action. On the other hand, when we feel safe and not under pressure, we tend to let go and relax; our breathing slows down and our eyes and ears become less sharply focused.

If you touch someone in the correct way, at the appropriate time and with the right attitude, the touch will soothe and support them. No doubt you have experienced at least a hand on your shoulder from the right person at the right time when you were upset. It helped, did it not? Conversely, that shove from someone who saw you as an object in their way made you feel irritated, and your muscles tensed up.

So, if you push someone, you can expect them to tense up and take up a closed defensive posture, or even an aggressive stance towards you. If you offer a supportive contact, such as catching someone as they trip over, their attitude to you is likely to be positive and this will be reflected in a lessening of their bodily tensions when they are interacting with you. Try leaning against a good friend in an appearance of being tired; they will instinctively support you. Then push them and see what happens! It is interesting that the Japanese written character for human suggests that to be leaned on rather than to be pushed is fundamental to human co-operation. It implies that benevolent human contact makes both us and those with whom we come into contact *more* human.

Shiatsu technique emphasizes this leaning, 'humanizing' principle. You always lean rather than push to apply pressure. In other words, pressure is applied using your body weight rather than with muscular strength. Exactly how you do this is covered in Applying Shiatsu Technique.

PREPARING TO GIVE SHIATSU

This chapter looks at how to set the scene for a successful
shiatsu session, which is as relevant to basic foundation level shiatsu
as it is to professional shiatsu therapy. It is not just a matter of arranging
your working environment but also involves preparing your body
and your mind.

Preparing your body: the Makko-ho positions

Shiatsu is normally given at floor level rather than on a couch or table, so the giver must be able to move around with ease on the floor. It is therefore important to keep your legs, hips, pelvis and spine supple. A system of exercises known as Makko-ho positions, which is practised widely by shiatsu practitioners and students, is designed to achieve this. In addition, the Makko-ho positions open each pair of channels, enabling you to monitor whether the Ki in any particular channel is blocked or weak. Both blocked and weak Ki will tend to manifest as stiffness during the exercise, although weakness of Ki can sometimes show as hyper-mobility accompanied by a sense of instability in those joints most closely associated with the movement. In other words, where a channel is more jitsu, the exercise will be difficult due to stiffness. For a channel which is more kyo, the exercise may feel stiff, or it may feel easy but a bit wobbly. Until you know exactly where the channels are, this nuance will not be so relevant. Appendix VI (page 128) gives diagrams of the channel locations for readers who wish to explore this aspect, but the positions are effective no matter whether you are familiar with channel location or not.

When doing the Makko-ho positions, try to remain relaxed throughout, except where stated otherwise; in some exercises I have indicated a part of the body which you should contract while relaxing the rest of your body. The following checklist applies to each position:

• Breathe in, then move into the position as you breathe out.

• Check that all your muscles are relaxed.

• Remain in the position and breathe in again.

- Exhale and try to let go a little more.

- See if you can passively allow yourself to relax a little further into the position.

- Never bounce or push yourself into the position; go very slowly and stop where it still feels comfortable.

- Do three or four long and slow exhalations while dwelling in each position.

- Carry out the exercises in the order given, because the effect of each position is designed to be enhanced by the previous one and to enhance the following one.

Don't worry if you fail to get very far into any position; it is the *intention without expectation* that counts here. All exercises from the sitting position tend to be easier to carry out if the buttocks are raised on a stiff cushion or block 5–10cm (2–4 inches) high.

The effects of these exercises are enhanced if you consider the emotional or psychological function of the channels affected from the perspective of Oriental medicine (indicated in italics). However, they will still be effective if you choose to ignore that aspect.

You can do these exercises at any time of day, but you will be stiffer in the morning than in the evening, so remember to take that into account. To minimize the risk of injury for readers who are not accustomed to doing exercises of this nature, I have made some minor amendments to some of the original Makko-ho positions, based on modern research into body mechanics.

Lung/Large Intestine

This exercise (see right) facilitates a more efficient *intake of Ki* by 'opening' the Lung Channel and enhances the ability to *let go* (both physically and emotionally) by activating the Large Intestine Channel. Go into the position very slowly and come up equally slowly. Keep your knees bent if you have slight problems with your back and avoid bending forward at all if you have severe back problems or very low blood pressure.

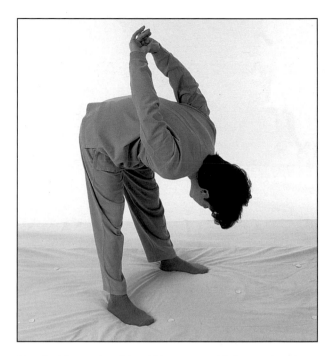

Stand with your feet hip-width apart and link your thumbs behind your back. Lean forward, dropping your head.

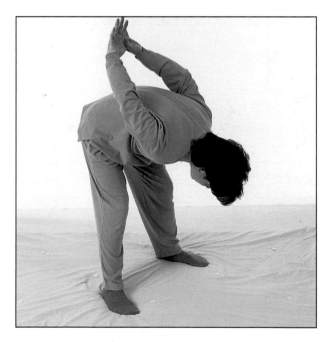

Stretch your hands away from your shoulder-blades rather than over and beyond your head. Keep your knees slightly bent unless you are used to similar exercises such as forward-stretching yoga postures.

Stomach/Spleen

These channels relate to our *desire to grasp food*. That could be why they are on the front of the body – when you're really hungry, you tend to go forwards rather than backwards to get food! Do not do this exercise if you have a problematic lower back or inflamed knees, and go down further than shown in the picture only if you have total confidence in your own flexibility. Below are two variations which largely eliminate potential strain on your lower back and knees.

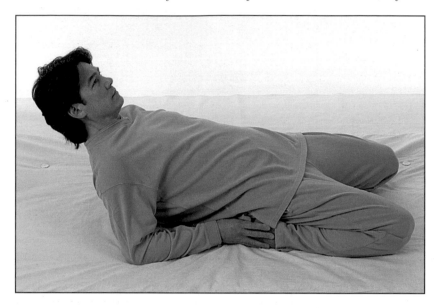

Kneel down with your feet tucked back and with your buttocks on the floor or on a cushion. Rest back on your elbows. Keep your buttocks as tightly clenched as possible to counteract potential strain on your lower back. Puff your chest out and keep your chin tucked in. Go back further only if you are confident in your own flexibility. Go down very slowly and come up equally slowly.

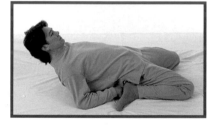

Your toes should be tucked beneath your buttocks; do not point them away from your body, as shown here.

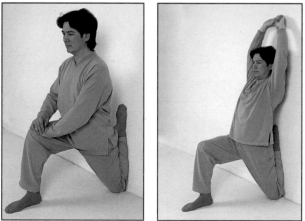

To eliminate potential strain on lower back and knees, kneel with your left knee against the wall, resting your buttocks against your heel. Your right leg should be bent at a right angle, foot on the floor. Contract your buttocks and bring your lower back towards the wall as far as is reasonably achievable. Lift your arms overhead if you want maximum stretch. Repeat on the other leg.

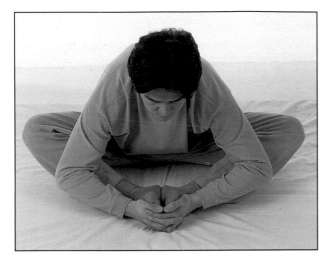

Clasp your feet in front of you as close to your groin as you can, with your knees spread apart. Curl forwards in a relaxed way, tuning into the feeling of 'inward attention'. Your elbows should be outside and in front of your shins.

Heart/Small Intestine

The Heart relates to our raw awareness or consciousness, whereas the Small Intestine enables us to assimilate mental concepts and information as well as food. This exercise involves folding yourself around your centre, which will naturally make you feel more *calm and centred*. It brings your awareness to areas on the inner surface of your body which relate to the Heart and simultaneously 'opens' the Small Intestine Channel.

Bladder/Kidney

This exercise 'opens' and 'frees' the back of the torso and legs, giving those areas sufficient Ki to ensure you can stand up straight and *go forward in life with confidence*. Do not pull on your feet or ankles, and bend forward very slowly and come up equally slowly. *Never force this position*.

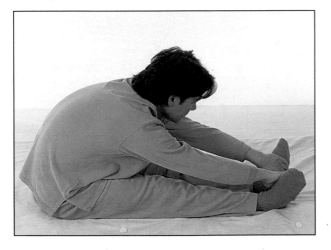

Sitting with your legs straight out in front of you, bend forward from your hips and place your hands, palms turned out, between your feet, with your little fingers uppermost. Aim your navel towards your thighs, not your head towards your feet.

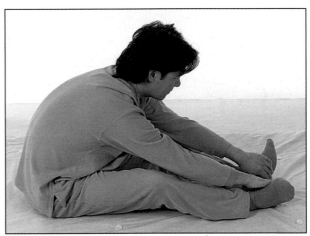

If you are particularly stiff in the hamstrings or have lower back problems, bend your knees a little and focus on any sensations you feel in the back of your legs. This will help activate the Bladder and Kidney Channels. If your legs can almost straighten, it may help to have your buttocks raised 5–10cm (2–4 inches) on a firm cushion or block. If you cannot reach your feet even with your knees slightly bent, hold your ankles.

Preparing to Give Shiatsu **23**

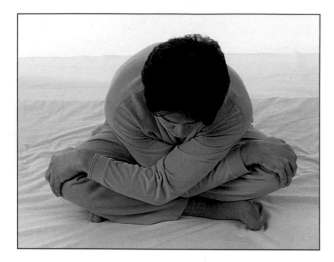

Heart Protector/Triple Heater

The Heart Protector protects the Heart both physically and emotionally, while the Triple Heater gives us a sense of *protection* against more general outside influences. Therefore, this enclosed Makko-ho position (see left) gives us a sense of our exposed outer shell (where the Triple Heater Channel lies) protecting our soft inner Heart Protector Channel. This position thus gives a general feeling of *protection and security*.

Sit cross-legged and cross your arms the opposite way. Exhale as you curl forwards. Reverse your arms and legs and repeat.

Gall Bladder/Liver

The Gall Bladder has much to do with our ability to make decisions, whereas the Liver gives the quality of *foresight* and the ability to make plans. Both channels are principally involved in keeping our Ki flowing smoothly. As such, 'opening' these channels, which involves a stretch to the side of your torso, activates an enhanced *decisiveness* about which direction to take in your life and in your day-to-day activities.

The order in which these exercises are done is in accordance with the Chinese channel clock cycle (see Appendix V, page 127). While you do not need to refer to this, do remember to carry out the exercises in the above order.

Sit with your legs spread as wide as you can. Stretch your right arm overhead and place your left arm across your ribs. Lean down towards your left leg, constantly drawing your right shoulder back and your left shoulder forward, while opening your chest as much as you can so that your back remains as flat as possible. Do not crane your head forward or bend your knees. Do the exercise slowly, with awareness and without strain.

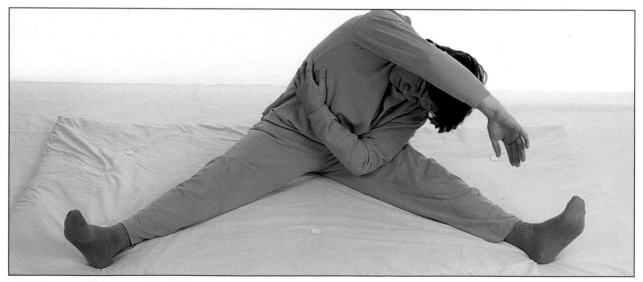

Do-In exercises for the hands and feet

There is a system of exercises for unblocking and strengthening Ki known as Do-In (Japanese) or Tao-Yinn (Chinese). Do-In includes a wide range of stretching, acupressure, rubbing and percussion techniques, but one simple aspect useful for our purposes here is a preliminary Do-In method used to keep the joints of the hands and feet supple and free of blocked Ki. In all cases, it is important to complete the exercises on both hands and feet. For the giver of shiatsu it is particularly helpful to keep Ki flowing smoothly throughout the feet and hands because free flow of Ki in the feet helps to keep the giver grounded while smooth Ki flow through the hands ensures a better touch sensitivity and greater potential for the transmission of 'healing touch'. These exercises are traditionally performed at dawn, but they can be done at any time. If you do them when you get up in the morning, an excellent way of starting is to run your hands and feet under cold water. Your feet especially will feel incredibly alive and warm afterwards as blood and Ki rush into them. This feeling of aliveness will then quickly extend throughout your whole body. Keeping a box of pebbles under your bed to walk on as soon as you get out of bed provides another good boost, providing a form of general reflexology 'tonic'.

You will be surprised at how much you can consciously influence the workings of your body if you can accept that Ki will go where your mind directs it. Therefore, if you clearly visualize stuck Ki leaving the wrist while fresh blood and Ki enter it, that is what will happen. The more finely honed your mental focus, the better this will work.

Do-In exercise for the wrist

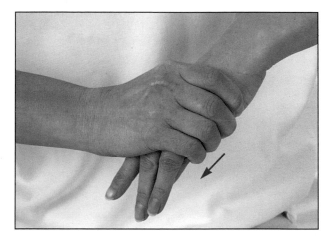

1. Apply a little traction to your wrist joint as you exhale then release it. Now flap your wrist, keeping it completely flaccid and holding an image in your mind of dislodging the debris or 'stuckness', expelling Ki stagnation and increasing blood flow, rather like drops of water spraying from a wet cloth from which you are trying to shake out excess water.

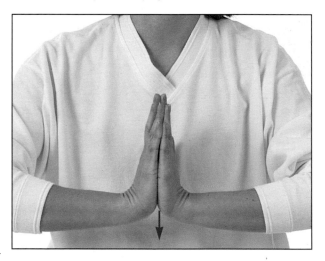

2. Hold both palms together in a prayer position with your hands held close to your chest and your elbows spread, thus extending your wrist joints. Move your hands down towards your waist until you feel the heels of your hands beginning to pull apart. Practise will result in your wrist flexibility improving so that you can bring your hands progressively further down. Imagine that all restriction to this movement melts away. You can then visualize clean oil working its way into all parts of the wrist joints.

Do-In for fingers, ankles and toes

The following set of illustrations show a series of similar Do-In exercises for the fingers, ankles and toes. Follow the same principles and visualizations as the example just described for the wrist. *Do not force any movement* in any of these exercises.

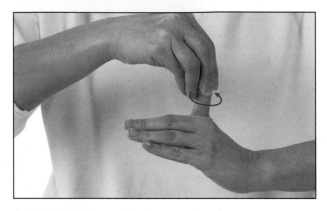

1. Take hold of your index finger and apply some traction to the finger as you rotate it. Rotate in both directions. Exhale as you apply the movement, visualizing increased blood flow and the expelling of waste products along with stagnant Ki. Repeat on all fingers in turn.

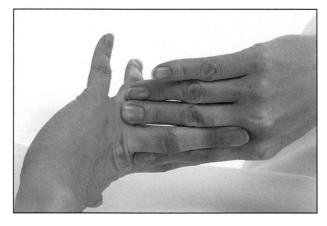

2. Make a fork with your index and middle fingers and lever each finger of the other hand in turn away from the palm, exhaling as you apply the movement. Imagine all restriction and stiffness melting away. Finish by flapping the hand and wrist.

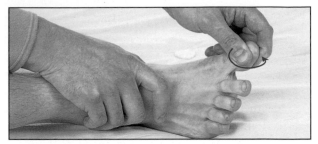

1. Take hold of your big toe and apply some traction to the toe as you rotate it. Rotate in both directions. Exhale as you apply the movement, visualizing increased blood flow and the expelling of waste products and stagnant Ki. Repeat on all your toes in turn.

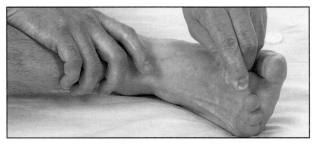

2. Gently lever each toe in turn towards the dorsum of the foot, exhaling as you apply the movement. Imagine all restriction and stiffness melting away. The third, fourth and fifth toes may even touch the dorsum of the foot within a few days of practice, but do not force them.

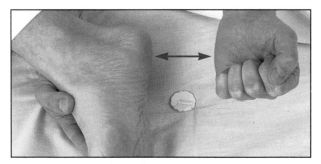

3. Beat the sole of your foot with your knuckles or fist for about 30 seconds. Be firm, but do not bruise yourself. Imagine you are beating the debris of Ki and blood stagnation out of the foot and ankle, thus dissolving all stiffness. When you stop, imagine you can feel all the pores in the sole of your foot breathing. Finally, stand on one leg and vigorously shake your other foot in the air. Imagine you are flushing out stagnation and poisons from your foot.

Your own wellbeing

The giver of shiatsu needs to work on his or her own health in as many ways as possible – you will not give such good shiatsu if you do not feel well. Also, because one tends to seek in others what one lacks in oneself, those with less vitality – less Ki – will tend to gravitate towards those with more vitality. So in order to attract people on whom to practise shiatsu you should try to be at least as healthy as they are. Ki tends to flow from the one with the greater supply to the one with the lesser supply, so you are not going to help the receiver of your shiatsu if your Ki is depleted in comparison to theirs – in fact, you could drain them of their vitality and cause them to feel a lot worse. Consequently, you have an obligation to your shiatsu recipients to keep your Ki clear and strong.

Most shiatsu practitioners practise some form of meditation, yoga, taiji quan or Qigong, all of which, if done correctly and with sufficient diligence, will improve one's Ki. Qigong is a Chinese concept, the correct meaning of which is 'any training or study dealing with Qi (Ki) which takes a long time and great effort'. In that sense, even shiatsu and acupuncture are forms of Qigong. However, in modern common usage it has come to mean 'practices which encourage Qi development in the body', such as taiji Qigong exercises. There are hundreds of Qigong methods, each with many variations; some emphasize stillness and internal visualization, some emphasize slow movement, and others involve sudden spontaneous movements. All are designed to reap long-term benefits resulting from long-term practice rather than being a quick way to feel good.

Hatha yoga asanas will 'open' and flush the Ki channels if they are done correctly, even if they are not taught specifically with Ki channels in mind. (Energy pathways akin to Ki channels are known as 'nadis' in yoga terminology.) Yoga is now extremely popular, and if you decide to

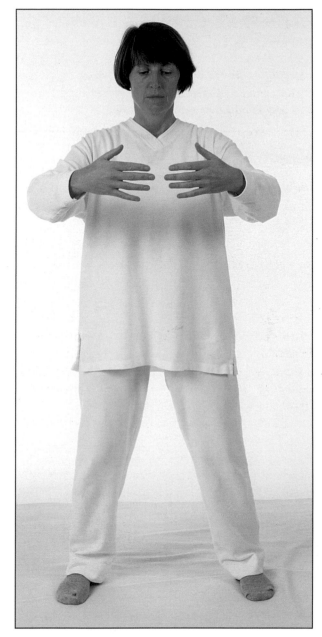

A standing Qigong exercise which is designed for calming the mind and grounding the body.

follow this route you should have no difficulty in finding classes locally.

Good old-fashioned exercise is great for maintaining and developing Ki, as long as it is non-destructive. By that I mean there is no point in damaging your joints in an attempt to build your Ki. The best exercises are those which encourage a full range of diverse movements that are not contrary to the way your musculo-skeletal system is designed to move. Walking, running (preferably over undulating terrain), swimming and so on are all excellent. The rules are:

• Moderate exercise smoothes and builds Ki.

• Excessive exercise exhausts and blocks Ki.

• No exercise at all tends to weaken your Ki.

Japanese Aikido masters often elect to tend their own land manually, as they consider the hard physical work involved helps to keep their Ki strong. This option may not be a practical one for you, but if you exercise regularly, work enthusiastically and sleep sufficiently, the quality of your Ki will have a head start. If you then do some deliberate Ki-enhancing activities, your Ki will improve and develop quickly. It must not be forgotten that moving around the receiver as you give shiatsu involves a degree of exercise. If done well, giving shiatsu will benefit your Ki. Done badly, it will block your Ki and cause you discomfort, if not immediately, then later on.

Nutrition

For every piece of advice on how to eat correctly there is a completely opposite view claiming equal legitimacy, and it can be confusing to know which regime to follow. I would suggest you avoid consistently eating junk food, but if you do so now and then, do not feel guilty about it. It is not what you eat on occasion that matters; what counts is what you eat as your staple diet. Even then, worrying about what you eat is likely to be far worse for you than actually eating it. Get some basic awareness of what foods are bad for you, make a deal with yourself to avoid them, then forget about it. If one day you succumb to temptation or absentmindedness and eat them, just accept the fact and forget about it.

Freshness is a good indication of a food's Ki level, assuming it has not been tampered with to give a false impression of freshness. To avoid that pitfall, eat organic food as far as possible. However, even when it is organically grown, if the food looks old and deficient in Ki then it *is* deficient in Ki, meaning there is less Ki for you to extract from it.

Burning food destroys it, leaving proven carcinogenic residues, so avoid burnt or smoked food. If you really want to be healthy, avoid that part of food that has been even lightly browned during cooking. A good motto is: 'If it's brown, put it down.' Water, when heated, exhibits strong Ki, so boiling or steaming your food is good. Cook it just enough to make it easier to eat.

Oils and fats are subject to the worst adulteration in the food manufacturing process. All the trace elements we require have been removed from commercial oils, and the balance of essential fatty acids has been altered; in their place are additives to make your bottle of oil neutral in taste and to extend its shelf life. Try to buy unrefined oils extracted from organically grown seeds and keep them in a sealed dark bottle or container in a cool place. Light, oxygen and heat destroy natural oils very quickly. For this reason, it is not good to cook with your oils and frying with them should be particularly avoided. If you do cook with oil, heat it within water to avoid raising the oil temperature above boiling point, which will tend to destroy most oils. Butter, and especially ghee from butter, can be cooked at a slightly higher temperature, but even that should be occasional rather than regular.

The closer a food is to its natural state, the better. Eat clear and wholesome food on a day-to-day basis and your Ki will be clear and wholesome. In short, eat Ki. Green leafy plants seem to have the most Ki, so eat all the edible parts in abundance. If you consume a cocktail of irradiated chemicals that have been burnt in your oven at every mealtime you will sooner or later not feel very healthy – so say goodbye to burnt, overcooked, overprocessed and stale food.

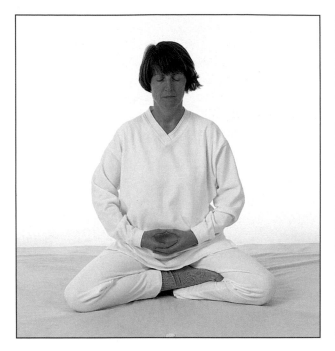

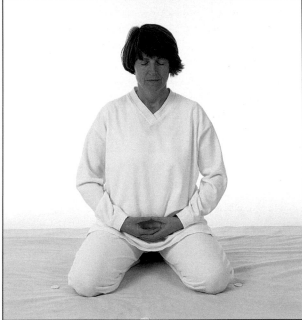

Preparing your mind

When you put your hands upon someone else's body, the actual mechanics of contact, such as the level of pressure and rhythm of movement, are essential ingredients for good shiatsu. However, this is not the only factor which will have a bearing on how your touch is received; your state of mind is also very important. Your attitude to the receiver, your reason for doing shiatsu, your emotional disposition and your ability to remain focused are all critical elements.

Mental focus

When applying shiatsu technique, be it a stretch or the application of pressure, you must be careful not to hurt the receiver. Conversely, you should not be so timid as to lack effectiveness. Often there is a fine line between overenthusiasm and inhibition, and the recognition of this line requires sensitivity. In its turn, sensitivity demands a focused mind.

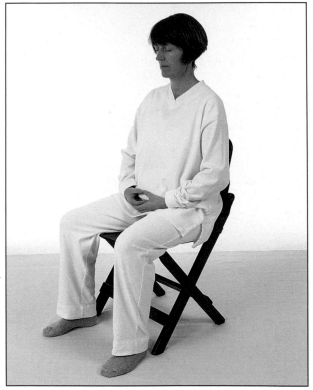

The photographs above show examples of correct postures for seated meditation. All require your back to be fully upright but relaxed.

If your mind wanders while you are giving shiatsu, you will miss the signals that indicate whether you should increase or decrease the pressure or stretch. One way of keeping your mind focused is to go slowly and ask the receiver to tell you when you are entering their 'discomfort zone'. However, because of the often extremely relaxing nature of shiatsu, the receiver may put up with moderate pain and not say anything until their pain is too much to bear. Shiatsu does not need to be painful, and if you are alert to the reactions of your touch you eventually learn to recognize the line between effectiveness and discomfort.

So how can you stay focused? First, you must work on your own body as already described to ensure you can remain comfortable throughout the session, for if you are experiencing discomfort you will be focusing on your own pains rather than on the receiver's reactions to your touch. Secondly, you would do well to practise a technique such as meditation, yoga or Qigong which trains your mind to remain 'one-pointed'.

However, a focused mind does not necessarily mean a compassionate mind. One can focus one's selfishness and hate as easily (if not more easily!) as one can focus compassion. You need compassion to develop empathy, and you need empathy to enhance compassion. Making a habit of reflecting deeply about the needs and suffering of others will enhance your caring attitude.

Mindfulness

To practise 'mindfulness' means to be constantly aware or 'conscious' of everything we do. It requires us to keep our minds absorbed in the present moment, noticing the detail of our actions. For example, if we wash a cup with mindfulness, we notice the texture and temperature of the cup. We are aware of how much pressure we are applying to the cup with the cloth or brush; we take note of the speed with which we are conducting the activity, and we become aware of our own physical sensations and thought processes.

The more repetitive or routine the activity, the more likely it is that we will switch to auto-pilot and allow our minds to dwell elsewhere. This is necessary in order for us to find time to make plans or to reminisce, but in our busy lives we perhaps spend too much time pondering the trivial, dwelling on the past or anticipating future possibilities. We thus tend to miss a full appreciation of the present. The past is history and the future is only a possibility; the only reality for us is what our consciousness perceives right now, so, if you wash a cup with your full attention, you will learn a great deal about that cup. By the same token, if you apply your shiatsu touch with your full attention, you will learn a lot about your touch and how it is received. If you make mindfulness a priority and a discipline, you will spend more time in the here and now. Consequently, you will learn a lot about yourself and about how you interact with others. Your shiatsu will naturally become more empathic and thus more effective.

One of the easiest ways to practise mindfulness is to observe your own breathing. A good technique is to observe the breath as it enters and leaves your nostrils, trying to notice any sensations felt at the point of entry and exit. You may feel this close to the tip of your nose, just inside the nostrils or between your nose and your top lip. Experiment to see which applies to you. Try to register only those sensations felt at this point; in other words, don't follow the breath deeper into the body on the inhalation, or beyond the nose on the exhalation.

Alternatively, be aware of your belly moving slightly in and out as you breathe, relating only to the sensation of your lower belly 'opening' a little as you inhale and 'closing' a little as you exhale. Again, avoid following the breath to see where it goes. These techniques are examples of a 'mindfulness of breath' method known as 'anapana'.

If you practise breathing with awareness, you will remember to do other things, including shiatsu, with more awareness. Do not be obsessive or obtrusive about it – just quietly continue until it is a natural part of your life. You will be pleasantly surprised at the benefits, particularly the way you are able to cope with stress more positively.

Meditation

Both mindfulness and anapana are examples of meditation. However, meditation encompasses any method which helps to counteract the wandering tendency of our mind so that we can experience a genuinely objective view of the world about us. The on-going awareness that things are both forever changing and ultimately interlinked with all other things is the reality which eludes us; we get fleeting moments of 'awakening' but then fall back into our habitually limited way of perceiving things. Take your own experiences as examples: when someone annoys you, you react angrily. Later, you might realize that the problem was your emotional overreaction to your own point of view. Such enslavement to your emotions will affect your shiatsu session. It will be hard to concentrate fully on your receiver if you are still smouldering with anger over some recent incident and you might apply a less sensitive touch, thus causing your receiver to suffer unnecessary pain.

The ultimate goal of the full-time meditator is to remain in a state of 'reality awareness' long enough to reach a full understanding of life and the universe. However, for both full-time and part-time meditators, the short-term benefits consist of: greater equilibrium and clarity of mind, leading to greater patience and tolerance; less stress, as seemingly stressful things are seen in perspective and therefore reacted to more positively; better health, because positive mental attitudes can heal physical and emotional problems; fewer unrealistic expectations of people or things, therefore less disappointments and better relationships; and a more realistic and positive self-image as the perception of reality broadens and deepens.

Types of meditation

There are two broad categories of meditation: stabilizing and analytical. The former consists of concentration exercises designed to settle the mind into a period of uninterrupted focus on a single point – the exact opposite of our usual state of mind, which is forever distracted. Mindfulness practices and concentrating on the breath are examples of this type of meditation; concentrating on a visualized image, a concept or a mantra are other examples.

Analytical meditations are periods when you consciously reflect upon and analyse a particular concept. The purpose of this method is to gain an understanding of how things are, to a depth which gives you enough clarity to convince you of the true nature of that concept. Initially you identify your erroneous conceptions. For example, if you are exploring compassion, you would aim to arrive at some insight into it by first eliminating your misconceptions about it.

Stabilizing and analytical meditations are usually combined within a single meditation session. For example, as you prepare to meditate on your breathing, as in anapana (a stabilizing meditation), it is helpful to spend a few minutes clarifying your state of mind and motivation for engaging in that session, which involves analytical thought. During both analytical and stabilizing meditations your mind will frequently wander, causing you to constantly bring your attention back to your breath as an anchor for your mind. At times it may be difficult to do this, at which time a return to a period of analysing your state of mind will help.

When you reach the point of intellectual understanding during a session of analytical meditation, let go of the thought process and focus your attention singly on associated feelings that arise. You will then arrive at a combined intellectual and experiential insight, causing your mind to become one with the object of your meditation.

Your level of success will depend on your depth of concentration, which comes through practice. Regularity matters more than quantity, because your mind is strongly influenced by habitual patterns. Start with 5–10 minutes and build up to 30 minutes, ending your session before fatigue and boredom set in. Don't push yourself too hard because as soon as it becomes a burden you won't do it. On some days you will experience more distractions and discomforts while other days you will be serene and focused. View the troublesome sessions as opportunities to explore and grow.

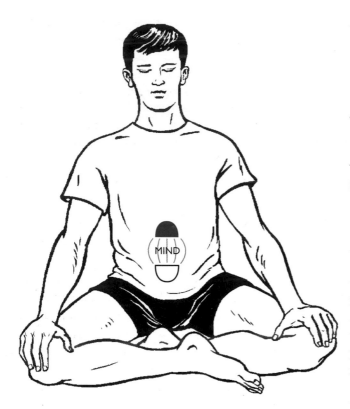

Active visualizations can help to focus the mind and to prevent sleepiness, restlessness, excitement and other distractions during a shiatsu session.

Meditation is not essential in order to practise shiatsu on your family and friends, but the more you do, the more it helps. At least employ 'mindfulness' during a shiatsu session. That is essential. Everything else is a (great) bonus.

Tips for successful meditation

Common problems experienced by people who are inexperienced at meditation include sleepiness, restlessness or excitement, and discomfort or pain which allows negative thoughts to intrude. The following are some simple suggestions for dealing with them.

Sleepiness

• Hold your spine straight, but not tense.

• Hold your head slightly forward, with your chin tucked in.

• If your eyes are closed, open them half-way and meditate with your gaze fixed on the floor some way in front of you.

• If you have an unexpected feeling of depression, remember that thoughts and feelings come in waves, so wait for them to pass rather than cling to them.

• If the room is dark, increase the light slightly.

Sleepiness antidote visualization

If the above suggestions fail to stop you wanting to doze off, try this exercise (left) before continuing with your session: imagine the bottom half of a large hollow white seed about the size of half a tennis ball in your belly 5 cm (2 inches) below your navel. Then picture the top half of a hollow red seed of similar size deep in your solar plexus. Imagine that your mind fills the space between the two seed halves. Now visualize the two seed halves shrinking as they converge just in front of your spine at the level of your umbilicus. As they do so, your mind becomes fully encapsulated within this tiny red and white seed. Next visualize a tube about a finger's width in diameter situated just in front of your spinal column, running from the base of your spine to the top of your head.

Finally, imagine the seed shoots up through that tube to emerge above the crown of your head. The seed evaporates, allowing your mind to expand into, and merge with, a vast empty void. Dwell upon this experience for a few moments before returning to your original meditation.

Restlessness or excitement

• Hold your spine straight, but not tense.

• Hold your head slightly forward, with your chin tucked in.

• If there is something particularly exciting in your life, reflect upon the fact that excitement is always short term. Feelings such as excitement come in waves, so wait for them to pass.

- If your breathing is too quick and too shallow, focus on your lower belly and observe your breathing as if it doesn't belong to you. Notice how it just happens without you having to exert any control over it.

- If the room is light, decrease the light slightly.

Excitement antidote visualization

Do the first part of the visualization for sleepiness up to the point where the seed halves shrink and converge with your mind inside. Dwell for a few moments on the feeling of centredness and groundedness created by the fact that your mind is now snuggled up inside a seed which is anchored deep in your belly. Then return to your original meditation.

Discomfort and pain

- Experiment with your position. If you are experiencing lower back pain, sit on a higher and/or firmer cushion. Lean up against something if necessary.

- If there is stress on your knee or ankle as a result of sitting in a cross-legged posture, put cushions under your knees, kneel in seiza (see page 41) or sit on a chair.

- If you are suffering from tension as a result of unresolved worries or anger, use the problem as a focus for your meditation. Also, imagine the pain evaporating from your body with each exhalation.

Pain antidote visualization

Imagine your consciousness as a gentle shower of cool water washing you down from head to foot, being fully aware of every part of your body as the 'shower' washes over it. Whenever your mind 'washes' into a painful area, imagine the pain is swept away. The hotter your pain, the cooler you should make your 'shower'.

If the pain does not go away, or become acceptable, just observe the pain and try to see it as merely another sensation. Alternatively, mentally increase the pain as much as possible before returning to the original pain, which should then seem less intense. If you can neither dispel nor accept the pain, stop the meditation and try again another time.

Negativity

- Bring your attention back to the breath, then use the negative thought as the object of your meditation.

Negativity antidote visualization

Imagine you are sitting neck-deep in a tub of warm water. As a negative thought arises, feel it soak out of your body (or out of the red and white seed behind your navel) into the surrounding water. When the water becomes discoloured by your negative thoughts, imagine the water emptying away so that all those bad thoughts disappear down the drain. The dirtier the water the better, because it means you are expelling more and more negative thoughts. Fill up the tub again, via an imaginary shower pouring onto your head. Repeat until no more negative thoughts arise and the water in the tub remains clean.

When negative thoughts arise during subsequent meditations, do the same visualization and feel you are washing out deeper and more subtle layers of mental debris. Avoid trying to repress feelings of negativity as they will only emerge again later in an exaggerated form.

A MEDITATION CHECK-LIST

- Make yourself comfortable in your chosen posture.

- Check and acknowledge your motivation and goal; it might be simply to calm down, perhaps so you can develop greater 'clarity' when you give shiatsu.

- Before you leave your meditation, recall your goal to see whether or not you fulfilled it.

- Allow much of what you have gained to spill over into your daily life.

- Dedicate your efforts and offer your gains to the welfare of others. This really helps to link your motivation for meditating with your real reason for doing shiatsu, namely to alleviate suffering.

Preparing your working environment

One of the advantages of shiatsu is that it requires no specialized equipment other than a mat and a couple of cushions. It is thus a very portable form of bodywork, though most professional shiatsu practitioners rent a room in their local complementary medicine clinic, work in specialized hospital clinics or set aside a room in their own home specifically for giving shiatsu. However, some do go to the receiver's residence or place of work.

If you are practising basic shiatsu techniques on family and friends the choice will be between their home and yours. If you do have to travel, leave plenty of time and practise mindfulness of breath on the way as you should not arrive stressed. From this point of view your own home is to be preferred, and there you can also arrange a suitable environment. A separate room used solely for shiatsu is the ideal. This is because the feeling within a defined space, especially an enclosed one, will gradually become influenced by the activities which take place there. If bitter arguments often take place in a room, that unhappy atmosphere will permeate the room. If, on the other hand, the room is used solely for shiatsu and activities such as meditation, yoga and Qigong, the room will take on the same peaceful feeling associated with shiatsu itself.

Creating an ambience of serenity in a room has many advantages. First, those who receive shiatsu in that room will react by starting to relax even before you begin working on them, so much of the preparatory work towards reducing their stress will have been done by the room itself. Secondly, when the positive ambience of the room builds to a sufficient level, the room will become akin to a sanctuary for you. You will find that upon entering the room to give shiatsu, the familiar feeling of serenity associated with that activity in that particular space will override any negative feelings you may have at that time. You will, in effect, have entered a 'bubble' which seems divorced from the normal stresses of life.

If you cannot set aside a whole room for shiatsu, try to reserve a space within a quiet room. A good ambience will still begin to manifest itself there, though maybe not so quickly or strongly, as the space is not exclusively devoted to shiatsu. If you cannot reserve a corner solely for shiatsu, at least try to give shiatsu in the same place each time; going to that familiar location will trigger your mind to switch into shiatsu mode.

The contents of your shiatsu room

Once you have established a location for your shiatsu sessions, what should you put in it? Not much! Material clutter will clutter your mind and that of your recipient. All you need is a mat about 2.1m (7ft) in length and 1.5m (5ft) wide, with enough room around it to apply your shiatsu. The shiatsu practitioner most frequently uses a shiatsu futon, which is a mat consisting of two or three layers of compressed cotton or wool within a cotton covering. The futon is 2.5–4cm (1–1^{1}/$_{2}$in) in depth, compressing a little with use. For hygiene, place a cotton sheet over the mat or futon and provide a small cloth or some soft paper about the size of a pillowcase to place under the receiver's head, particularly for the face-down position. Have three or four fairly firm cushions nearby so that you can support the receiver's head and limbs when required.

Lying in a cold room would not be much fun for the receiver, so make sure the room is warm and in addition provide a blanket to keep them especially cosy once you have finished. The only other thing you might need is a lightweight cloth about 75cm–1m (2^{1}/$_{2}$–3^{1}/$_{4}$ft) square to place between the receiver's skin and your hands when you are working on their neck or face, especially if their skin is sweaty or greasy.

Judicious placement of plants will enhance your room and you could perhaps hang a few simple pictures on the wall, but nothing too evocative.

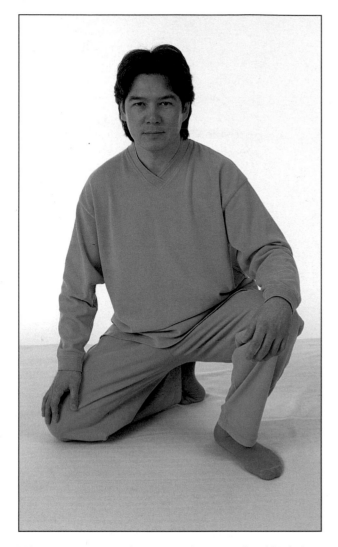

When you are giving shiatsu wear loose, comfortable clothing made of natural fibres.

You may want to include art and decor which reflects the inner you, but expressing your personality is not the point in this particular room – you have the rest of your house in which to do that. The shiatsu space must be as neutral as possible. Remember, you want to create your 'bubble' to be independent from the rest of your life's ups and downs.

Keep your working space clean, simple and welcoming. Beyond that, you could consider the feng shui (energetic configuration) of the room and either read one of the many books that are now available on the subject or call in a feng shui practitioner.

Finally, should you play music while giving shiatsu? Shiatsu does not need the presence of music, so this is very much your choice. However, bear in mind that music can be very evocative. The musical track which may engender serenity in you could remind your recipient of an unhappy or even traumatic incident, so check first that your recipient will find it equally soothing.

Clothing

The receiver of shiatsu should remain fully clothed throughout the session. A single layer of cotton or some other natural fibre is best because shiatsu feels better and less obtrusive through a barrier of thin natural fibres. Most synthetic fibres seem to make it more difficult to feel the quality of the tsubo. If you apply shiatsu directly to bare skin it tends to be more superficial in its effect, because the sensation of skin contact distracts the giver from feeling the deeper and more subtle presence of Ki. The sensory nerve endings are most prolific on the skin surface, so a cloth barrier will dampen down the surface tactile sensations and allow the receiver to experience a deeper connection. Although it might seem that a tsubo would be easier to find and feel on bare skin, a little practice through clothing will reveal this to be untrue. To reduce the likelihood of any sexual connotations arising, it is best to encourage the receiver to wear loose-fitting clothing.

For the giver of shiatsu, loose-fitting clothing made of a natural fibre is also the preferred option. You need to be able to move around without restriction, and feel well ventilated around your joints. To avoid unnecessary contact between your clothing and the receiver, there should be no dangly bits such as belts, tassles or untucked shirt hems. For the same reason that it is not a good idea to make your shiatsu room an extension of your personality, avoid dressing to make a statement. The more your ego takes a back seat, the easier it is to feel what is happening to the receiver.

APPLYING SHIATSU TECHNIQUE

Shiatsu technique should never come from muscular strength. Instead, it should utilize gravity wherever possible, which is to say that the giver should lean rather than push or pull.

In order to lean correctly, you need to be aware of your centre of gravity, which is located in your belly, or 'hara', as it is called in Japanese. If you ensure that your movements originate from your hara they will involve the whole of your body, thereby utilizing the sum total of your body's power.

It is well understood in the martial arts that if, when throwing a punch, the practitioner focuses mind and breath in the hara and pivots from the lower belly, the weight and power of the whole body will be behind that punch. If the punch originates from the shoulder it uses the power of the shoulder only, which has only a fraction of the

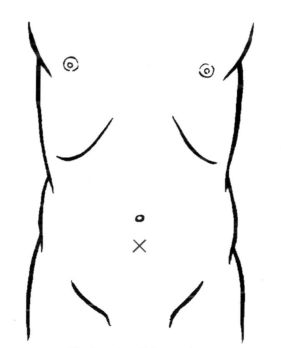

The location of the tanden

power that originates from the hara.

Using your hara therefore means that you originate all your movements from your belly, or, to be more specific, from a point in your lower belly just below the navel, which is the body's central pivotal point. This point is known as the 'tanden'.

So, whenever you perform a shiatsu technique, you must ask yourself, 'From where in my body does the movement originate?' By working backwards from the point of contact you can use 'mindfulness' to detect the source of your pressure or connection. If you are performing the technique correctly, the source will always be discovered to be at the tanden, in the lower hara.

If you want to apply pressure upon the receiver's back with your palm, for example, and on working back from your palm, you find that the root of the technique is a push from the shoulders, then you will know the technique is not correct; it is not rooted in hara and is therefore ineffective. Not only that, it will most probably create a defensive reaction in the receiver rather than the relaxation response that you are trying to achieve.

The broader meaning of hara

However, the meaning of hara extends beyond mere physical movement; it is a term that is used to illustrate one's ability to achieve. If someone applies themselves diligently to fulfil their aim, they are said to have hara. Whether they actually achieve that aim or not is considered a reflection of how strong in hara they are. How one accepts disappointment in not achieving one's aim is also a reflection of hara. That is, the ability to lose with grace and start all over again with undiminished resolve and effort indicates a good hara.

As such, to have hara means to have the ability to get things done; to not shy away from the difficult and to bounce back after setbacks. So to have a strong hara in shiatsu practice will make your shiatsu more effective on all levels: the techniques will come from a source of relaxed power, and your motivation and ability to keep doing shiatsu will be assured.

Focusing energy in the hara harmonizes the body, mind, emotions and spirit, which enables us to harmonize with our surroundings and to react positively to the needs of those receiving shiatsu from us. When someone is described as 'coming from their hara', the meaning is that they are well grounded, strongly focused and using the maximum potential of their body and mind together.

So it is essential that you develop power and focus in your hara, but just how do you set about doing that? The answer is that you keep active, stay humble, do a lot of shiatsu from your hara and focus your mind frequently upon your hara. You could also practise anapana hara focus (see page 30).

Why babies give good shiatsu

If you observe babies as they move about and play you will be able to see that their movements originate from their centre, their belly. You will never see young babies tensing in the shoulder to push a toy, for example. If you can persuade a baby to crawl about on your back, you will be able to experience the key qualities of shiatsu contact: the complete surrender of weight to gravity, giving the quality of 'weight underside'; movements and balance centred in, and emanating from their belly; and an innocent non-analytical acceptance of themselves being there, not invading your space.

A baby's mind, when drawn to an object, will for a while become completely absorbed and preoccupied by that object. During that preoccupied period, their mind is completely 'one-pointed', totally focused. Their consciousness is not yet cluttered and their sense of self is not so separated from their environment. They are thus able to be completely in the present and to relate to the object of their attention as if it is part of themselves.

The shiatsu practitioner tries to recreate those qualities. We need to be a little bit 'innocent' to be aware of the receiver's needs; to lose our sense of self in order to empathize with the other person. Babies empathize perfectly; they are just limited in their variety of means to express that empathy. Adults empathize less perfectly, but have great powers of language to hide their lack of communication abilities.

When we occasionally get a glimpse of what the world was like when we were more innocent, we realize just how colourful and rich things really are. To touch another's body with innocence and clarity means we will realize how much more is going on within that person. This is so simple, yet so difficult. It may be largely a lost art for the adult, but it can be at least partially regained by observing and contemplating life and by giving attention to preparing your body, your mind and your working environment (see Preparing to Give Shiatsu).

Cross patterning

When we crawl we put one hand forward as we place the opposite knee forward. This leads to a well-balanced and co-ordinated means of getting around. Try crawling by putting the left hand and knee forwards at the same time and see what happens! When you have an opportunity to watch a baby stretch a hand out, notice that their opposite leg moves also – and notice how both the arm and leg movement connects at their hara.

Research has suggested that inhibition of this diagonal limb movement, which is called 'cross patterning' or 'cross crawling', inhibits the correct integration of our analytical thought patterns with our more intuitive or experiential thought processes. This implies that it is better for both our physical and mental balance to ensure that when we apply pressure through one hand or fore-arm during a shiatsu session, we also involve some participation with the opposite leg.

Whether you have your hands on the floor or on a person makes no difference to this principle. Therefore, if you practise this exercise as you apply those shiatsu techniques requiring down-ward pressure through your hands (see Prone Sequence), you will soon learn how to develop your hara as you practise on your friends.

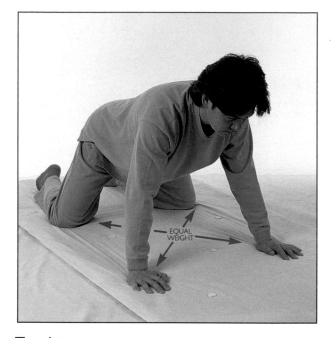

Try this exercise:

1. Kneel on all fours as if you were about to crawl but with your hands and knees spread a little wider apart and further from your torso, with your weight balanced evenly between your hands and knees.

What if you lean forwards and apply equal weight through both hands? If you forget about your legs and concentrate only upon your hands, you will feel the root of the technique coming more from your shoulders. If you do the same technique but concentrate on the sensation of connecting to the ground with your knees, you will feel the root of the technique in your hara.

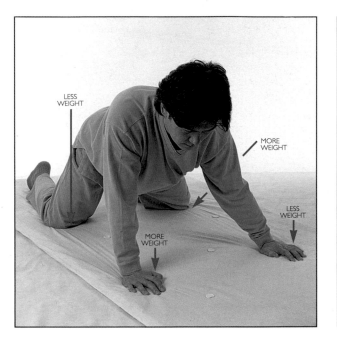

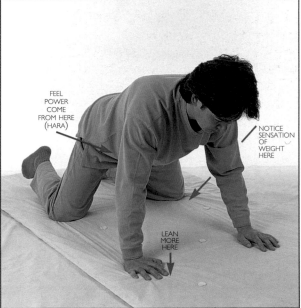

2.   Lean more weight through your right hand by shifting your hara slightly towards your right hand. Notice that you feel a slight increase in weight through your left knee. (If you did not clearly feel that diagonal weight distribution between hand and opposite knee, lean well forwards onto both hands and try lifting your left hand off the ground so that the right hand is supporting most of your weight. You will notice that it is much easier if you also lift your right knee off the ground so that it is your right hand and left knee supporting your weight.)

3.   With your belly completely relaxed and 'open', lean more weight through your right hand as you take the weight off your left hand, without actually lifting your left hand off the ground. Then consciously allow your left leg to feel as heavy as possible so that your left knee feels more heavily pressed into the ground, simultaneously taking the weight off your right knee. If you focus your attention on your hara as you do this, you will feel a sensation of gathering power within your hara. Even out the weight distribution between all four limbs and repeat this exercise several times to appreciate the difference it makes.

Basic shiatsu stances

There are several basic positions or stances from which to apply shiatsu technique. Stances fall into three broad categories: kneeling and squatting; sitting; and standing. Most stances used in the Foundation Course are drawn from the kneeling and squatting section. More advanced shiatsu techniques sometimes require different stances, but they fall outside the scope of this book.

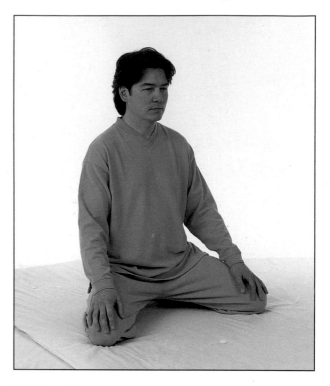

Wide kneeling

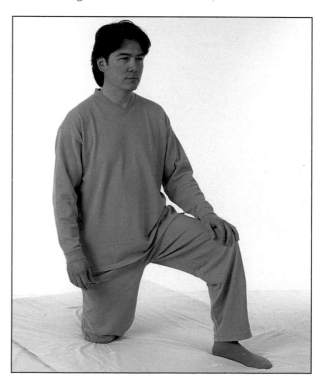

Half kneeling

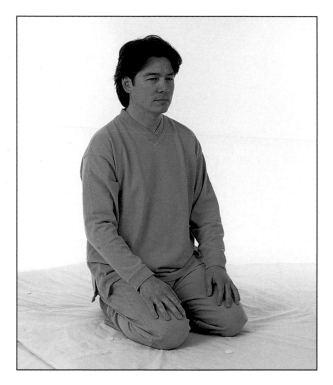

Kneeling or seiza (sometimes called 'kneel sitting')

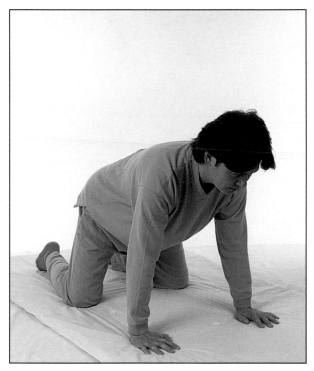

Prone kneeling

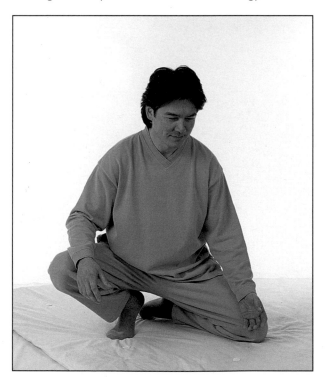

Squat kneeling

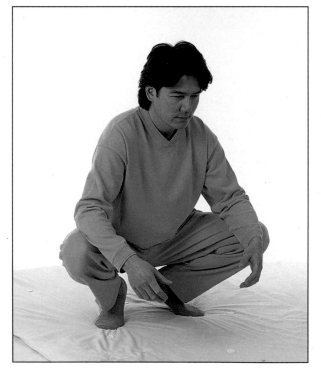

Squatting

The correct posture for giving shiatsu

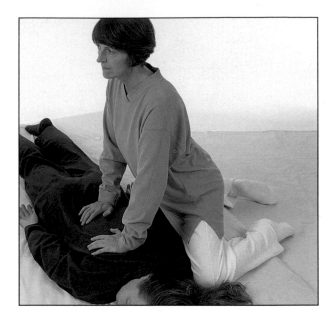

Correct posture: the head is straight and the eyes are looking straight ahead; the back of the neck is open and lengthening; the shoulders are relaxed, with the shoulder-blades descending; the chest is open and the hara is open and relaxed; the base is wide.

It is important to hold your posture correctly while giving shiatsu as it will make it easier for you to support the receiver's body without fatigue. In addition, it will help you to move around their body more efficiently and will generally help your Ki to flow smoothly.

The basic rules of good shiatsu posture

• Adopt a wide base with your legs to ensure a low centre of gravity (any of the shiatsu stances described on pages 40–41 will do).

• Keep your hara relaxed and open.

• Look ahead, not down at the receiver (apart from an occasional glance to check that the receiver is comfortable).

• Keep your shoulders relaxed, feeling that your shoulder-blades are moving down your back, away from your ears.

• Keep your chest open, without forcing it.

• Feel the back of your neck is open, lengthening and relaxed.

• Imagine that the spaces within the joints of your spine, shoulder, elbows, wrist and fingers are constantly opening as they relax more.

When using your hands to apply shiatsu technique, it is important to ensure that your knee or knees are not positioned between your hands. You need a clear 'view' from your hara to the area you are working on, otherwise it is more difficult to apply your weight and to project your Ki or 'intention' from your hara.

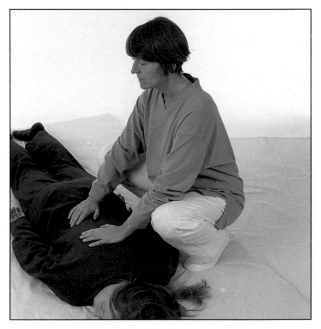

The correct knee position in relation to the hands while squatting, showing the knees spread to keep the hara open.

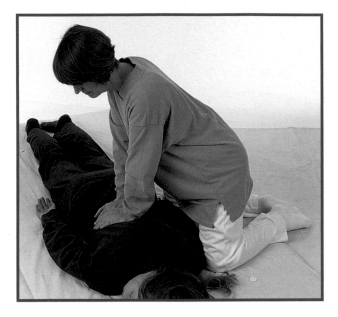

Incorrect posture: the giver is looking down, the shoulders are tight, the chest and hara are closed and the base is narrow.

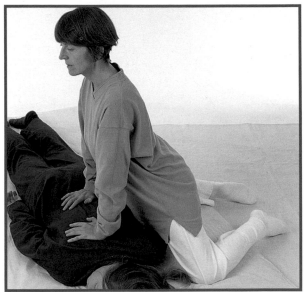

Incorrect posture: the lumbar curve is exaggerated, producing potential for weakening the lower back.

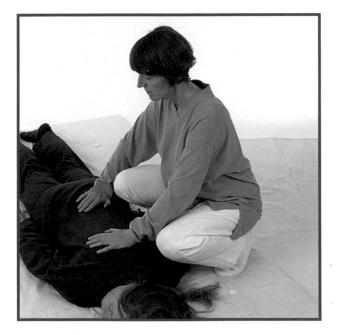

Incorrect knee position with the knee between the hands, blocking the hara.

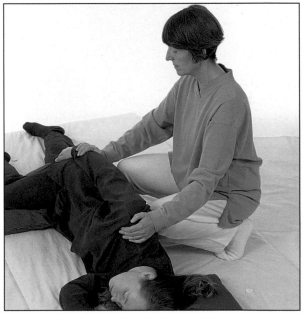

The correct knee position while squatting when the knees are used to apply shiatsu technique. The knees are between the hands and the hands are spread wider to ensure balance and control of pressure from body weight.

Applying Shiatsu Technique **43**

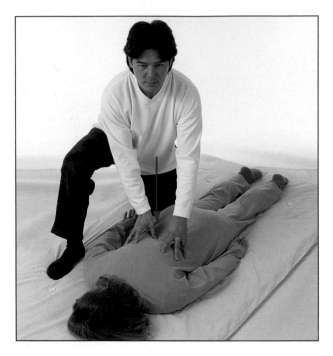

Tsubo on receiver's body and an imaginary 'eye' positioned on the giver's hara, aligned such that the eye can see directly down the neck of the tsubo.

Positioning your body in relation to the receiver

When giving shiatsu it is important to make sure that your hara is aligned with the area upon which you are working, or to get as close to that ideal as is practicable without sacrificing your comfort. In other words, the more you relax your body when applying pressure, the more your body weight will naturally manifest onto the area you are working and the more your Ki will connect with the receiver.

Connecting your Ki simply means aligning your intention with your action, which is to say taking the most direct route to accomplish your goal. For example, when you are hungry, you turn to face the refrigerator and walk directly towards it; you would not walk in a round-about way to reach the food. Your hara points the way because your hara contains the source of power to reach your goal. In this example, the urge to eat represents your intention. Your mind initially mapped out the route to the refrigerator, and your hara followed that route so that you ended up at the refrigerator door. That one-pointed thought leading to direct action can be considered as an example of Ki projection, which is an aspect of what is called 'connection': First you had the idea; the mind then led your Ki towards its goal; your Ki then enabled you to fulfil your goal.

Where it is practicable you should align your hara to get the best 'view' down the 'neck' of the tsubo. One way of ensuring your optimum position is to imagine there is a rail running through your hara from the tip of your sternum (breastbone) to your lower belly; then imagine that you have an eye which can move up and down along this rail but can only look straight ahead. If you position yourself so that the eye can see down the neck of the tsubo to its base, you will be in a good position to apply technique to that tsubo. More experienced practitioners may not adhere strictly to this rule, but for beginners it ensures maximum effect while keeping the rules simple and minimal.

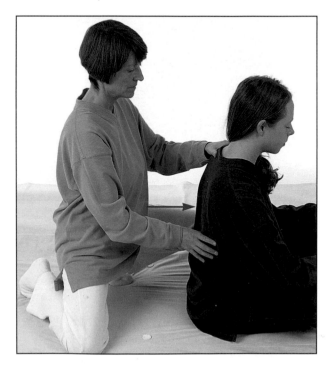

The hara aligned with the area of the body upon which you are working.

Applying the techniques

No special equipment is required to give shiatsu – different parts of your body are the only tools you need to apply the techniques. The part you use depends upon the type of connection and pressure you wish to give. At foundation course level, open palms, thumbs, forearms and knees are the predominant 'tools'. Experienced practitioners will sometimes use their hands in different ways to apply specialized techniques.

Palm techniques

The palms are the main tool used in foundation level shiatsu. Although less specific than the use of thumbs or fingertips, the palms have a more soothing quality. If a friend is distressed, we are naturally inclined to place a palm on their shoulder as a gesture of support, rather than lean a thumb into their back! The palms are icons of interpersonal communication, as illustrated by the gesture of shaking the hand of someone you meet.

The Heart Protector Channel (sometimes called the Pericardium Channel) terminates in the palm (see appendix VI). One of the subtle functions of the Heart Protector is that it enables us to share warmth and close communication with another individual. In a way, it acts as the avenue for spreading our consciousness throughout our body. The fact that the Heart Protector flows into the palm means that when we touch someone, we can give a 'conscious' touch. It enables us to transmit friendliness.

The Ki of the Heart Protector (your warm, supportive, healing quality) exits the body from the centre of the palm, at a point called Heart Protector 8 or 'Laogong', located at the place where the tip of your middle finger lands when you make a fist (see below left).

The whole surface of your palm should be kept in full contact with the recipient so that your hand can mould around the contours of their body. The palms will therefore lie more flat on their back, or curl to envelop an arm or an ankle. The palms and fingers must remain relaxed. The arms should remain outstretched, but with the elbows unlocked (see below).

When closer body contact is required, it may be necessary to have your arms bent at an angle of 90 degrees at the elbow, with the knee or inner thigh supporting your upper arm (see page 46). However, this will cause a slight reduction in the connection of Ki flow between your hara and your palm.

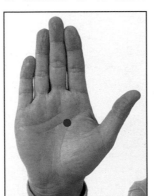

The location of Laogong in the palm of the hand.

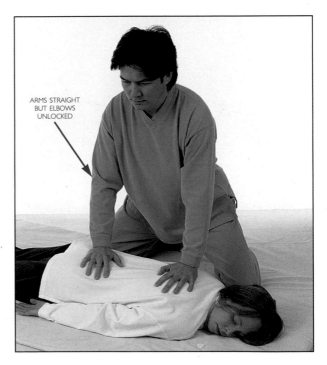

ARMS STRAIGHT BUT ELBOWS UNLOCKED

Applying palm pressure to the receiver's back with the elbows outstretched but unlocked.

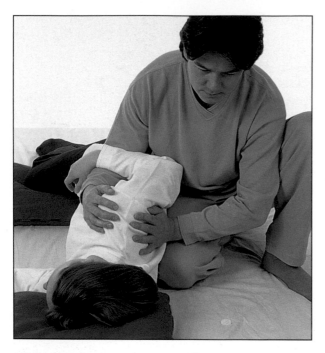

For closer body contact (see page 45), it may be necessary to bend your elbows at a 90 degree angle and support your upper arm with your knee or inner thigh.

Support hand technique

Keep both hands separated but in contact with the receiver. This is the most basic yet most important therapeutic shiatsu technique. It enables the giver to 'listen' with one hand while the other hand is engaged in techniques to tonify, calm or disperse Ki. The listening hand is often called the support or mother hand, while the active hand is sometimes called the working or child hand. When tonifying, the working hand should be applied at right angles to the area of contact. Dispersing techniques are any active techniques such as shaking, rubbing, circling and, especially, stretching. Calming is an attitude rather than a technique: if you are very calm and composed, that calmness will influence the receiver's Ki at the point of contact.

Palm overlap technique

Place one hand on top of the other. This technique can be used when a malleable wave-like action is required.

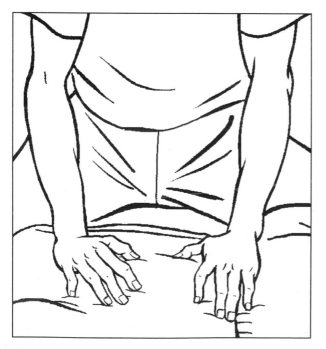

The support hand is on the receiver's body and the working hand is applied at right angles to the area of contact.

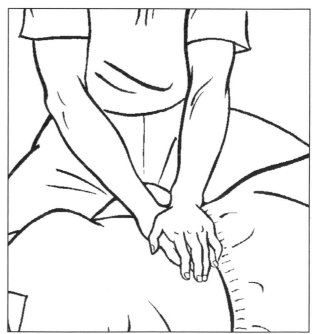

In palm overlap technique, the hands are placed one on top of the other.

Circular rotations

With one palm moulded into the contours of the shoulder-blade, buttocks or sacrum, firmly rotate the connective tissues over the underlying bone rather than merely scrubbing the surface. The other palm can be positioned either nearby on the body or on top of the other hand. Rotations are especially effective for relieving muscular tensions around the shoulder-blades or for stimulating warmth in the pelvic region when applied to the sacrum.

Shaking

Place the palm in the same way as you did for rotations, but shake it instead of rotating it. The effects are similar.

Grasping

One hand clasps the limb for support while the other moves along the limb. Also, both hands can clasp a limb as you stretch that limb away from the space between your hands.

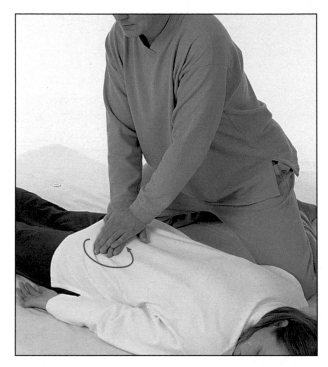

For circular rotations, the giver's hands can be placed one on top of the other.

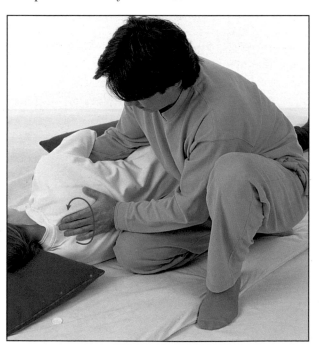

An alternative method for circular rotations involves the giver placing one hand on the receiver's shoulder and the other on the shoulder-blade.

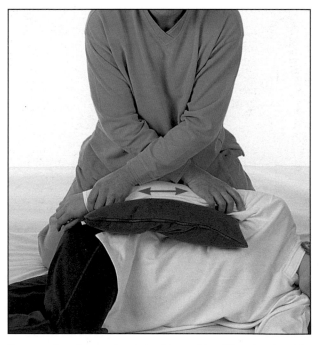

For grasping, the receiver is in side position. The giver has his arms crossed and both hands clasp the receiver's arm.

Applying Shiatsu Technique **47**

Double palm squeezing

Interlock your fingers and apply a squeezing movement simultaneously with the heels of both hands. This method is useful for squeezing the muscles either side of the lumbar spine from the kidney region down to the pelvis.

Palm off the body method

Holding the palms a short distance away from the body has a warming effect if the giver is relaxed

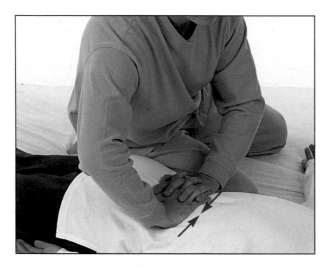

With the receiver in prone position, the giver is applying double palm squeezing to the lower back with the heels of both hands.

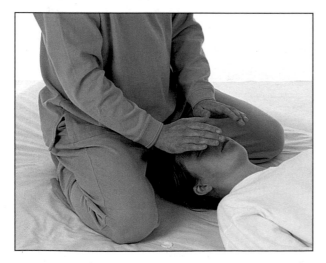

Holding the palms just off the body has a warming effect.

and centred. This method is especially effective when applied over the face, which can be a pleasant way to conclude a session. When Ki sensitivity is developed, local excess or deficiency of Ki can be clearly assessed using this technique.

Thumb techniques

The thumb is the classic tool of shiatsu and some styles of shiatsu use it almost exclusively, although this is very limiting; one tool rarely suffices for a range of variable situations.

As the thumb is shorter and thicker than the other fingers having only one interphalangeal joint instead of two, it is the strongest individual digit. Powerful pressure can be applied and sustained by the thumb if necessary. The ball of the thumb is used for most applications, although the area near the tip can be employed when working with light pressure between small muscle groups such as exist in the neck.

Some people have very flexible thumbs that will bend backwards when pressure is applied through them. If your thumb is of this type you run the risk of overstraining the interphalangeal joint and should minimize the use of your thumbs and make more use of the palms or fingers.

It may be that you will have difficulty keeping your thumbs straight, allowing them to buckle at the interphalangeal joint. If you apply strong pressure like this over a period of time, you will damage your thumb joints. Even light pressure given with buckled thumbs is discouraged. This is because Ki moves in straight lines or smooth curves; it does not make sharp right-angled turns. Therefore, if your thumbs are buckled, you will both feel less and give less through them.

There are two main methods for supporting your thumb pressure: the open hand and the closed hand. Two other variations of thumb application, the thumb adjacent technique and the thumb overlap method, enable greater pressure to be applied. However, such heavy pressure is unnecessary if your awareness and Ki is accurately focused on the kyo areas.

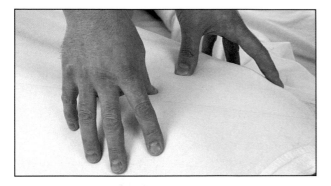

Open hand method applied to the receiver's back.

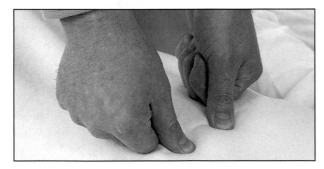

Closed hand position with fists supporting thumb.

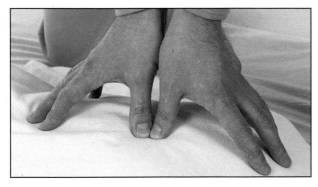

Thumb adjacent method with open hand support.

Open hand method

For maximum stability it is preferable to have your thumb in contact with the receiver's body and your other four fingers spread lightly in contact as shown left.

Closed hand position

Alternatively, the four fingers can be formed into a fist so that the thumb can be supported against the index finger. This method is a useful alternative for those with hyper-mobile interphalangeal joints, but it does sacrifice stability compared to the open hand method.

Thumb adjacent method

The thumbs are placed side by side, either in open hand or closed hand configuration.

Thumb overlap method (with open hand support)

Here one thumb is placed directly on top of the other. The weight is given more through the top thumb, allowing the lower thumb to be more passive. The open hand method with fingers spread lightly to each side can be used for support.

Thumb overlap method (with closed hand support)

As described above one thumb is placed directly on top of the other, but support is achieved by a closed fist resting on the receiver's body.

Thumb overlap method with open hand support.

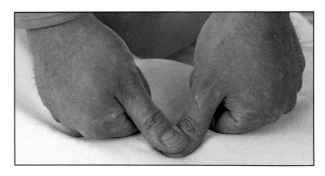

Thumb overlap position with closed hand support.

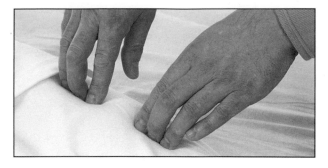

Three fingers of each hand tracking the Stomach channel in the thigh.

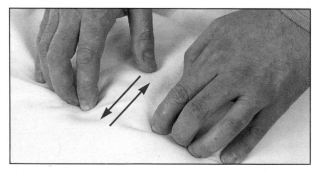

Four fingers of both hands doing 'kenbiki' technique for dispersing the muscles close to the spine.

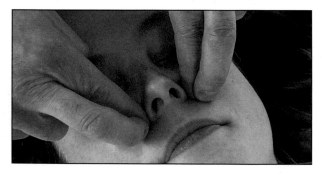

Index finger method.

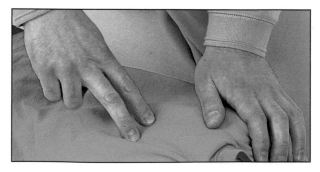

'Vee' finger technique.

Finger techniques

The fingertips are excellent tools for sensing the Ki within the channels and feeling other subtle activity registering near the surface of the receiver's body. This is because the fingers have a rich supply of sensory nerve endings. (Please make sure you keep your fingernails short – you will feel nothing through them, but the receiver will certainly feel something if you dig your fingernails into their body!)

Three- or four-finger method

Using the middle three fingers simultaneously is a good method for tracking along a Ki channel to find the kyo and jitsu discrepancies within that channel. Professional shiatsu practitioners also use three fingers of each hand to feel for kyo/jitsu patterns in the hara. It is an excellent technique for tonifying the spaces between the ribs, close to the sternum (breastbone). Placing all four fingers of one hand on the receiver's mid or upper back and circling or shaking them can be an effective way to disperse tension in the intercostal muscles between the ribs.

A two-handed version of the four-finger method can be used to disperse tension in the muscles close to the spine, using a to-and-fro 'push-pull' movement known as 'kenbiki'. Your thumb should be relaxed and your fingers strong (constant practice will quickly strengthen them). Like all shiatsu techniques, the movement must originate from your hara, with a sense of connection to tanden. This will prevent fatigue and tension accumulating in your wrist.

Index finger method

This technique is a useful alternative to the thumbs for people with hypermobile thumb joints when applying pressure to the side of the receiver's nose.

'Vee' finger technique

The middle and index fingers are lightly pressed simultaneously either side of the spinal column in small children.

Finger/thumb combination techniques

Dispersing claw technique

The thumb and fingers are slightly curled to form a claw. The claw is then pressed into the body and quickly withdrawn, as if pulling strands out of the body. In reality, excess Ki is being pulled out of the area being worked on. This technique is specific for pulling accumulated Ki (jitsu) from the shoulder-blades or buttocks. It is never to be used on kyo areas, as this will make an area that is already deficient much more so.

Tonifying claw technique

The position here is similar to the above, except that the fingers and thumbs are less spread. The thumbs are completely straight and the fingers are only slightly curved. This is particularly good for working down both sides of the spine at the same time in either the sitting or face-down position. The thumb is positioned to one side of the spinal column and the fingers are on the opposite side.

Dragon's mouth technique

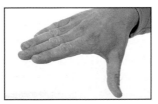

Spread your thumb and index finger wide. Contact is applied through the 'vee' shape. The 'dragon's mouth' is used primarily to apply pressure to the occiput. Both hands can be used together to apply pressure to the waist in the side position. The dragon's mouth can also be applied to the limbs, in which case the fingers are bent to give a stronger contact.

Baby dragon's mouth technique

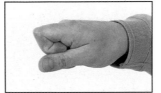

Make a fist, but with your thumb and index finger positioned as shown above and right. Like the tonifying claw technique, this technique is used mainly for working down both sides of the spine at once (see right) in the sitting, side and sometimes face-down position.

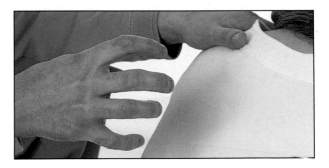

Dispersing claw technique on the shoulder-blade.

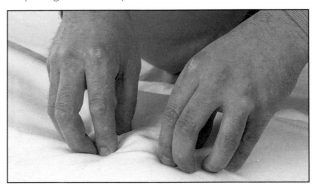

Tonifying claw technique using both hands down centre of the back with the receiver in face-down position.

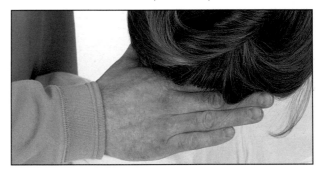

Dragon's mouth hand configuration.

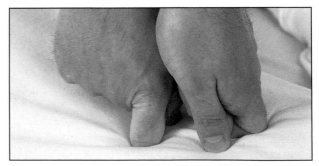

Baby dragon's mouth hand configuration.

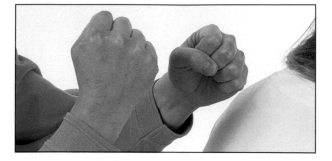

Pummelling with loose fists.

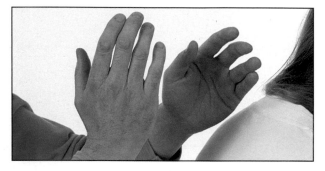

Loose finger chopping

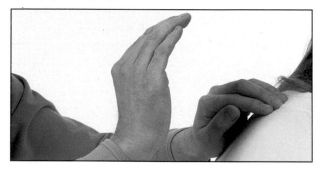

Palm cupping

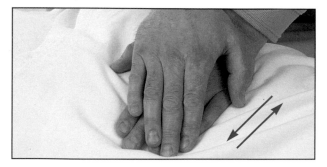

Rocking (very gentle rocking is suitable for recipients depleted in Ki, but more vigorous rocking should be reserved for those of a more jitsu profile).

Other hand techniques

Other hand techniques are occasionally used to disperse jitsu areas, as well as to increase blood and lymph to the skin and superficial muscles. These techniques have a very localized effect and are therefore subsidiary to the mainstream techniques. Used by themselves they are fairly superficial in effect. Even so, beginners should not apply these techniques to chronically ill people because they will be weakened still further if their Ki is dispersed too much. Therefore, except in specialized circumstances, these techniques are best reserved as useful adjuncts for loosening up robust recipients, especially in the sitting position.

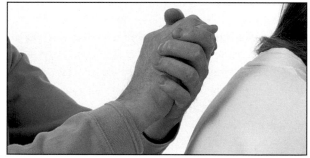

Double hand cushioning

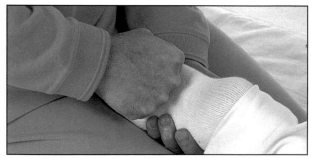

Knuckle rolling applied to the receiver's feet in prone position.

Forearm and elbow techniques

The area of your forearm close to your elbow can be used to apply strong pressure to the back, hips and feet. The forearm, or both forearms together, should be applied only after the area to be worked on has been palpated by the hands. This is because they are far less sensitive than the hands.

Single forearm technique

One forearm applied to the sole of the foot gives a great feeling of ironing out tension in the foot. Make sure your wrist is totally relaxed. As usual, all the pressure must come from leaning, never from pushing.

Double forearm technique

Use both forearms together on the back to stretch it. The forearms can also be used on the buttocks or thighs.

Elbow techniques

The elbows can be used on the same areas of body as the forearms when a stronger and more focused pressure is required. An acutely flexed elbow gives the strongest pressure, which in most cases is too much; a more open elbow joint angle gives a more comfortable pressure. It is essential to keep the wrist relaxed and fist open. You should not use your elbow until you have developed a high level of sensitivity with other 'tools' such as your palms.

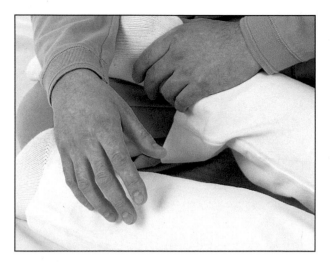

Single forearm technique applied to the sole of the foot.

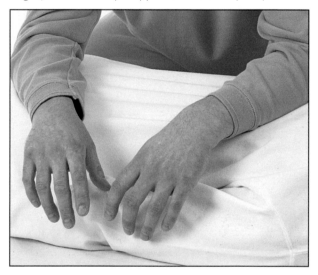

Double forearm technique applied to the back.

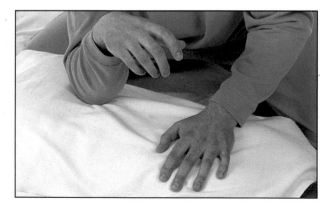

Elbow technique applied to the back at an acute angle.

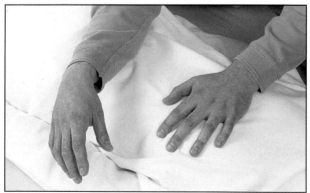

Elbow technique applied to the back at an open angle.

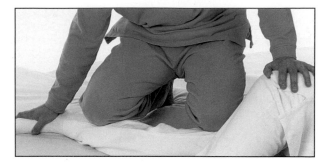

The knees on the inner thigh in side position.

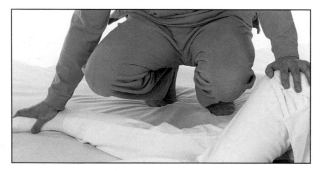

The weight is taken through the hands as the knees are lifted off the thigh.

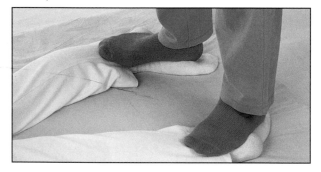

The feet can be used to stand on the ankles.

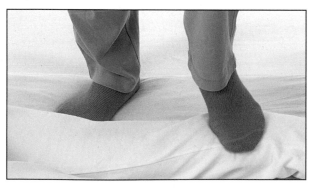

Shaking the foot on the calf muscles. Avoid the knee joint.

Knee techniques

Although you can develop great knee sensitivity by constantly practising techniques with them, they will never be as sensitive as your hands. Consequently, use them with discretion only on areas that have been previously checked by your hands. Your knees can be applied individually or together and you can give very firm pressure with them.

Keep both hands on the receiver's body so that your body weight is supported through your hands rather than through your knees. In other words, to ensure the receiver's comfort and your own stability, your hands must be placed so that you can instantly remove your knees if necessary.

Feet techniques

Your feet can be a very useful tool for shiatsu. Although less sensitive than the hands, because they spend most of their time in contact with the ground they can give a very 'earthy' quality to a session. If you intend to use your feet for shiatsu, walk around in bare feet as much as possible to give them an even greater earthy quality. Qigong will give your feet a feeling of connection with your tanden (your lower belly), improving your balance. You can further enhance this quality by imagining your feet are being filled from your tanden with sand or other heavy substance.

The feet can be used to stand on the receiver's ankles, which helps tonify the kidneys. However, they are used more extensively for temporarily dispersing jitsu areas in the limbs by employing a rapid shaking technique with light pressure. This can be useful for dispersing excessive tension on the surface when it is masking underlying kyo, thus rendering the kyo more accessible to palpation by hand. However, you must check that the receiver's ankles are flexible enough. Apply light downward pressure onto their heels with your hand. If the space between their instep and the floor disappears and there is no pain in their knee, then the technique is considered safe. Do not stand on their heels. Your toes should be on their ankles and your heels should be on their soles. Get feedback from the receiver at every stage.

Two-hand connection

The techniques which have the most profound effects upon the receiver's Ki are those which involve having both hands in contact with the receiver's body. The hands are your most sensitive Ki imbalance detectors and Ki projectors, so it stands to reason that two should be twice as effective as one. Two hands are even more effective if they are separated while in contact, rather than one overlapping the other. If performed correctly, the two hands separated method will result in the receiver experiencing both places of contact as one single unified area. This gives a deep feeling of the whole body being involved in the process. The body and mind will 'open' and relax because the receiver's parasympathetic nervous system will be activated. Conversely, a single point of contact gives only a localized soothing or dispersing effect, which may be appropriate for more superficial, local relief of pain or stiffness but does not have the same potential for addressing the Ki at the core level. To get away from a purely mechanical touch and develop the most conscious touch, do the following:

• With two hands separated and in contact with the receiver, focus your mind on your hara rather than on your hands.

• Sense that your hands 'begin' in your hara. You can do this by focusing on your inhalation and exhalation, as if you are breathing through your lower belly (see page 30).

• Tune into the sensation that your arms and hands are 'breathing' in unison with, and as an extension of, your hara.

• Now feel as if your total body breathing includes the part of the receiver's body that lies between your hands.

Once you have achieved this, you will experience both yourself and your recipient as part of the same 'circuit'. If your focused awareness can be sustained, you may sense the receiver's whole body as one integrated breathing, living unit. You might even feel yourself 'as one' with the recipient. A very sensitive practitioner can sometimes sustain this sensation when one hand is stationary and the other hand is moving, which greatly enhances the quality of continuity.

This level of awareness takes a considerable amount of practice, so do not despair if nothing happens when you try this for the first few times. At foundation course level, very profound benefits of two-hand connection will still be there whether or not you, the giver, actually experience these Ki sensations. It is simply a question of fine tuning your effectiveness with diligent practice.

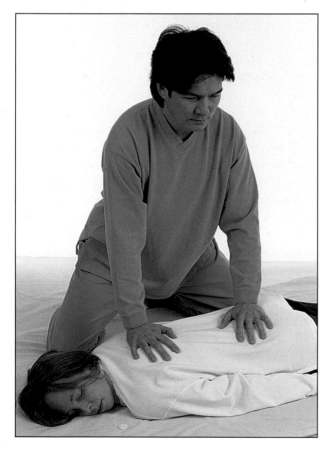

With two hands separated and in contact with the receiver, focus your mind on your hara rather than on your hands.

Two-hand connection along a Ki channel

When working to balance kyo-jitsu within a Ki channel, two-hand connection is essential. This level of work may begin at foundation course level, but becomes more central to shiatsu practice from the next level of study onwards.

In the practical application of two-hand connection, one hand will assume a more supportive or Yin role and the other a more working or Yang role. In either role, the part of the hand used can be the palms, thumbs or fingertips. However, the support hand mostly makes use of the palm.

The basic technique is as follows:

1. The support hand remains stationary on one part of the Ki channel, preferably a more jitsu part, while the active hand works down another part of the channel.

2. If the working hand is on a jitsu area, you either move it onto a kyo area or you apply techniques to disperse the blocked Ki from the jitsu area. (A dispersing technique is any active technique such as shaking, circling or stretching.) Meanwhile, the support hand 'listens' for the effects generated by the activity of the working hand.

3. If the working hand is on a kyo area, apply stationary perpendicular pressure (pressure applied at right angles to the area of contact) and wait for a reaction between the two hands. Often you will sense some activity in the kyo area through the working hand, or in the jitsu area through the support hand. The best result is to feel both, which indicates that the two areas are interrelating. A feeling of 'opening', then 'filling up' in the kyo area or tsubo is ideal, especially if accompanied by a feeling of yielding and emptying in the jitsu area.

4. If no response is felt after about 30–60 seconds, you can allow your support hand which is over the jitsu area to become the working hand and apply some dispersing techniques to that jitsu area. Sometimes this will 'shake up and wake up' the blocked Ki, inspiring some of it to move towards the kyo area.

By working in this way, you are coaxing the Ki to move from where it exists in excess to where it is deficient. If you can move the Ki from a jitsu area into a kyo area, as in step 3 described above, you will have succeeded in dispersing a jitsu area or tsubo as the direct result of tonifying a kyo tsubo. This is the best, deepest, most long-lasting and painless method. It is much better than just dispersing the jitsu without addressing the kyo. If you get the desired response during step 3, dispersing techniques such as shaking, circling and stretching are superfluous. However, if you do not get the desired response, you can use the dispersing techniques to coax things along a bit, as in step 4.

So, in effect, two-hand connection is the method to draw Ki along the Ki channels, in so doing smoothing out the Ki distortions within that channel. The effect of this will spill over into other channels, helping to regulate the body/mind functions in general.

Moving the Ki from the hara

Because the storehouse of Ki is within the hara, the object of shiatsu is to get your receiver's Ki to move from their hara through the limbs and into their hands and feet. For this reason, the support hand should be positioned closer to the centre of their body as the working hand gradually progresses away from the support hand and thus away from the centre of the body. In other words, the hands should start closer together and move apart rather than start apart and move together. However, no more than one joint should be between the support and working hands because joints interfere with clear communication between the hands. You can feel the Ki with one joint in the way, but it is very difficult with two.

The support hand and working hand should be applied with equal awareness to ensure total communication and consciousness of Ki flow between your hands. This is sometimes interpreted as equal pressure. For beginners, equal pressure is quite a good rule, although as your sensitivity develops, the actual equanimity and level of pressure becomes less important.

Offering maximum support and connection

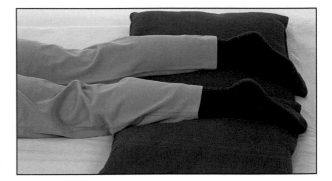

Cushions placed under the receiver's insteps when face down can make stiff insteps or knees more comfortable.

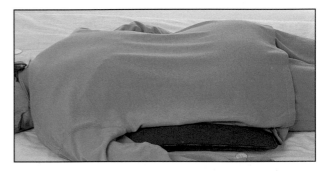

Cushions placed under the receiver's belly when face down may help relieve those with lower back problems.

Support has four aspects or meanings within the context of shiatsu, called 'levels of support'. The first level is to assist your recipient rather than imposing yourself and your shiatsu upon them so they will feel secure, trusting and at ease. If you are cold, indifferent or overbearing, they will not drop their barriers and may even feel aggressive towards you. Therefore, the first level of support is one of 'supportive attitude'.

The second level of support is to ensure physical stability for the receiver, so that they remain in position when you are working on them. The most stable position for the recipient is to lie flat on the floor, either face up or face down. In this position no muscular tension is required to offset the effect of gravity, which is forever trying to pull us onto the floor anyway. Ensuring your recipient's physical comfort also falls into this second level of support. In this regard, the judicious use of cushions for comfort and support can make a great deal of difference. For example, when they are in the face-down position you might want to place cushions under their feet to support their instep, especially when applying techniques to their lower legs. Lying face down can aggravate a weak or tender lower back because the lumbar spine feels compressed. This can sometimes be offset by placing one or two cushions under the receiver's belly to 'open' their lower back.

MAINTAINING A FLUENT CONTINUITY OF TECHNIQUE Adequate connection and support within good shiatsu technique will enable the recipient to experience a feeling of integration throughout their body and mind as long as the giver of shiatsu can maintain continuity. In order to achieve that:

• Apply your shiatsu session in a co-ordinated, flowing manner rather than as a disjointed amalgam of random techniques. The technique sequences (pages 62-119) exist to give you a framework to work within and if you keep practising them, your mind will become free of the burden of deciding what to do next. Later on, when you are fluent in technique, you can be much more spontaneous and innovative in your shiatsu sessions.

• Each technique should be a logical extension of the previous one and wherever possible contact should be maintained as your hands glide from one position to the next, so keep your hands in contact even when moving down the receiver's arm, leg or back, or changing technique. Making and breaking contact continuously will inhibit the receiver's ability to relax deeply because they will be unsure where your hand will land next.

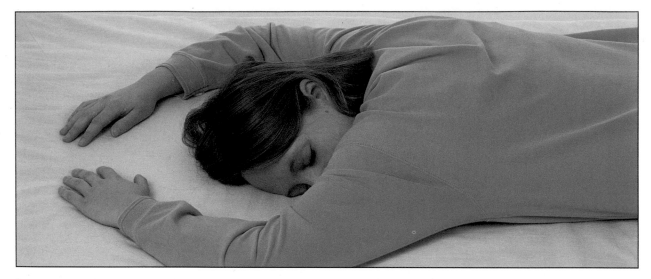

Some receivers find it more comfortable to position their arms beyond the head when lying face down.

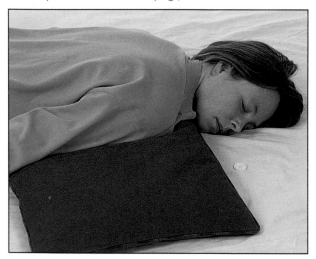

For a stiff neck when turning to one side in the face-down position, place a cushion under the corresponding shoulder.

Perhaps the biggest problem with lying face down is that many people cannot get their neck into a comfortable position. Lying with the head turned to one side is the most relaxing position if the neck is flexible enough. Those with stiff necks often try to lie with their nose on the mat which, even if they are able to breathe, will eventually cause fatigue in their upper back and neck. People with slightly stiff necks may still be able to lie with their head turned to one side if they place their arms on the floor beyond their head. However, this does make it more difficult for the giver to get into the Bladder Channel tsubo around the nape of the neck and upper back. From that point of view it is better if the receiver has their arms down by their sides, but their comfort is the prime consideration. If it is uncomfortable for them to lie with their head turned to one side or the other, try placing a cushion

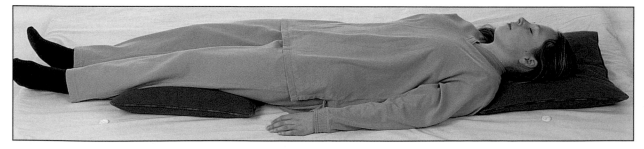

A cushion placed under the knees can ease knee and lower back problems, while a cushion under the head can help relieve the pain of a stiff neck.

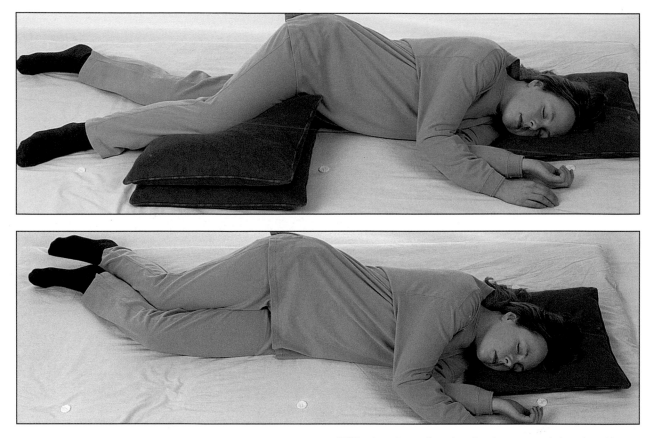

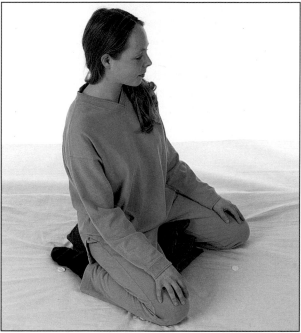

TOP: *A cushion placed under the receiver's head and knee when she is in side position can make the hip and head more comfortable and will help prevent over-straining the neck.*

ABOVE: *Alternative leg position, especially good for those who tend to collapse onto their front.*

A bolster between the legs makes kneeling more comfortable.

underneath the shoulder on the same side that the head is turned to, in order to take the strain off their neck. For those who can afford it, there is a system of moulded body support cushions designed to provide maximum comfort for the receiver, particularly when they are lying face down.

When lying face up, some receivers, particularly those with certain back problems, will feel more comfortable with cushions placed behind their knees. Those with round shoulders and/or stiff necks may be more comfortable with a cushion or pillow under their head. However, some people actually prefer to lie completely flat on their back

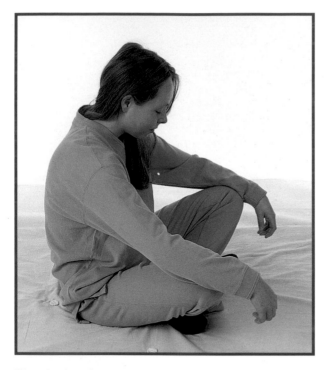

Tilting back in the cross-legged position can be uncomfortable.

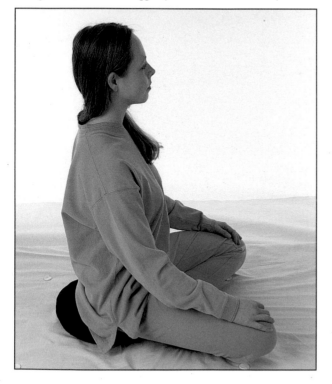

The receiver more upright in the cross-legged position, with a firm cushion under her buttocks.

with no supporting cushions. In the side position you should support the receiver's head with a pillow and position their legs in such a way as to prevent the receiver from rolling onto their belly. Sometimes it helps their comfort to have a cushion under their knee.

In the sitting position, some receivers prefer to kneel while others like to sit cross-legged. You can make kneeling more comfortable for some people by placing a firm bolster between their legs to take the pressure off their thighs and insteps. However, if the receiver is comparatively tall this may make them too high for you to apply shiatsu from a kneeling or squatting position and too low for a standing one. If the receiver prefers to sit cross-legged they will naturally be lower to the ground, which is an advantage for the smaller practitioner. Some people cannot comfortably sit cross-legged because their pelvis tilts too far back, causing lower back fatigue, in which case seat them on a thick, firm cushion or a firm foam block 6–10cm (2½–4in) deep. This will tilt their pelvis forwards and take the strain off the lower back.

The third level of support is the supportive touch. The receiver may react defensively if you push or press, but by initiating your movement from hara, and leaning rather than pushing, your touch will be welcomed rather than repelled. The recipient will therefore open and relax rather than tighten and close.

Finally, the fourth level of support is to be accessible if the receiver needs to clarify any after-effects arising out of their shiatsu session, in which case a supportive dialogue will put their mind at ease. This is more relevant for professional practitioners who are treating people with more serious problems. At this grass-roots level, where you will be giving general shiatsu for stress reduction, it is rare to invoke any uncomfortable after-effects.

The well-prepared session

Dressing for shiatsu:

* *Shiatsu not only feels better when received through a single layer of cotton or other natural fibre, but such clothing will also enable the giver to move freely and to feel well-ventilated around the joints.*

* *Clothing that is free of any tassels, belts etc. helps avoid any unnecessary contact between giver and receiver.*

* *Long sleeves are preferred as direct contact with the skin can distract the giver from sensing the presence of Ki.*

Mental preparation:

* *The giver has warmed up physically with a series of Makko-Ho positions and is now prepared for moving freely around the receiver at floor level.*

* *The giver's state of mind has an important bearing on the receiver. Qigong exercises have helped her ground her body and clear her mind ready for a focussed session of shiatsu.*

Correct posture for giving shiatsu:

* *The giver is looking ahead rather than down at the receiver.*

* *Her neck, shoulders and chest are open and relaxed.*

* *Her knees are spread to keep the hara relaxed and open.*

PRONE SEQUENCE

You are now ready to practise basic technique sequences or 'forms'. If the receiver is new to shiatsu it is best to start in the prone position as she will feel less 'exposed' than she would if she were lying face up or sitting. Make sure she is comfortable by placing cushions where necessary.

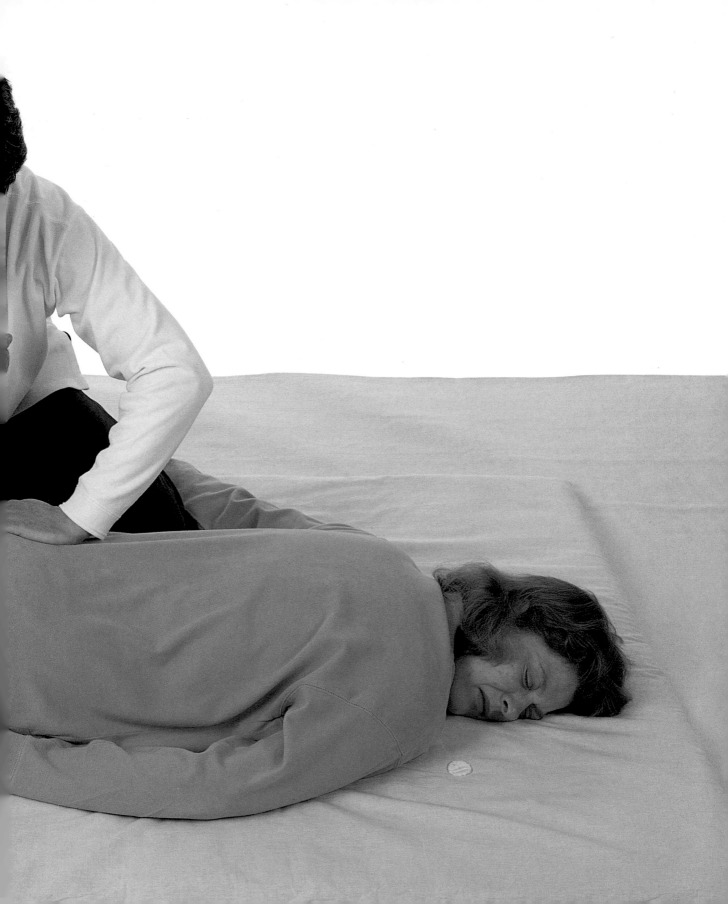

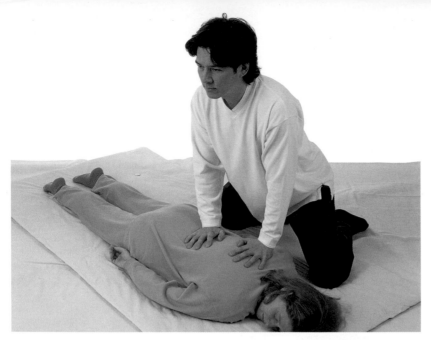

Baby walking

Kneel next to the receiver, ensuring you spread your knees wide enough to give you a low centre of gravity and thus a solid base from which to apply the technique. This position is known as 'wide kneeling'. Keep your head up and your hara relaxed and open. Lean forward onto all fours, leaning your body weight through your hands and 'walking' your hands randomly over the receiver's back and buttocks, like a baby crawling. Allow gravity to determine the level of pressure rather than applying pressure through pushing. Relax your hands and allow them to mould into the contours of the receiver's body. Avoid leaning the heel of your hand directly on her spinal column and do not lean too heavily on her lower back. You can extend the technique to the back of the receiver's thighs, but *do not* lean into the back of the knees.

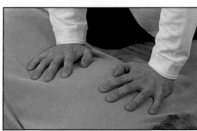

Relax your hands to allow them to mould into the contours of the receiver's body.

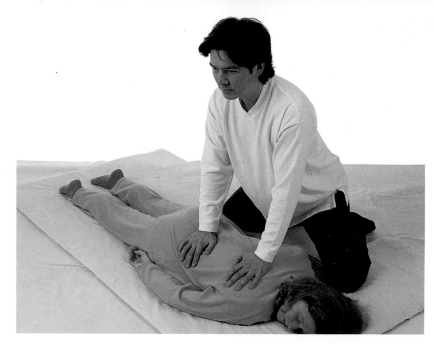

Palming

Maintain the same stance and posture as in Baby Walking (see opposite). Keep one hand stationary on the side of the receiver's back furthest from you, with the heel of that hand between her spine and shoulder blade. Use your other hand to palm down the back and into the buttock in a line just beyond the far side of the vertebral column. This area of the back relates to the Bladder Channel, which in Oriental medicine theory has an influence on the nervous system. This technique will therefore help to calm your receiver in a very direct way.

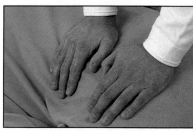

1. Rest one hand between the spine and shoulder blade as you palm down the receiver's back with the other.

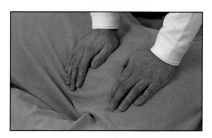

2. Keep the palming hand in a line just beyond the far side of the spine.

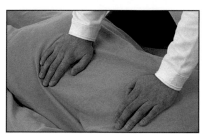

3. Palm down the length of the back, towards and into the buttock.

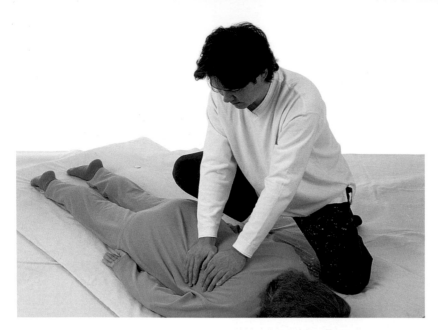

Stretching muscles away from thoracic spine

This technique is great for relieving stiffness in the upper back. There are two main versions to choose from. Maintain the same stance and posture as in 'Baby Walking' (see page 64). Place both hands on the far side of the receiver's upper back, with the heel of both hands in the natural groove close to her spine. Keep your belly and shoulders relaxed and lean forward, allowing some of your body weight to transfer through your hands into the receiver's back. As with all shiatsu techniques you should never push but where possible let gravity do the work for you.

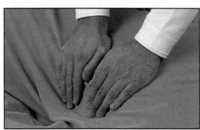

VERSION A

Allow some of your body weight to fall into the receiver's back simultaneously through the heels of both hands, thus stretching the muscles away from the spine. Synchronize your leaning forward with the receiver's exhalations.

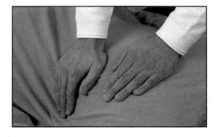

VERSION B

Instead of leaning through both hands simultaneously, shift your weight from one hand to the other so that as the weight increases through one hand it decreases through the other. Do not break contact.

NOTE DO NOT USE THIS TECHNIQUE IN THE LOWER BACK; THE VERTEBRAE OF THE UPPER BACK (THORACIC REGION) ARE ABLE TO ROTATE ALONG THEIR VERTICAL AXIS, WHEREAS THE VERTEBRAE OF THE LOWER BACK (LUMBAR REGION) CANNOT. TRYING TO DO THIS TECHNIQUE IN THE LOWER BACK MAY STRAIN THE LIGAMENTS AROUND THE VERTEBRAE.

Moving to the other side

While there are other methods of moving around the receiver, this way is good for developing fluency of movement and hip flexibility. When you have followed the sequence through, you will be ready to repeat the palming technique from the other side of your receiver, having successfully completed a 'transition'.

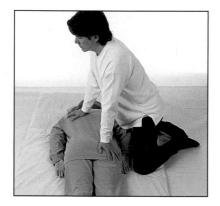

1. Place one hand on the receiver's nearside lower ribs or buttock. Place your other hand on the far side scapula (shoulder-blade).

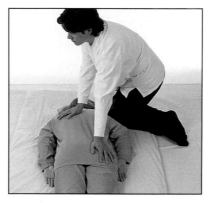

2. Position your leading knee so there is enough space between your knee and the receiver's nearside shoulder for you to place your trailing knee.

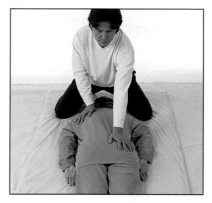

3. Now move your leading knee to the floor on the other side of the receiver's head, leaving sufficient room for the trailing knee to be placed.

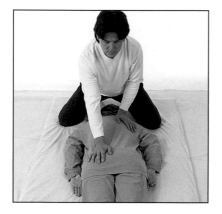

4. Glide the hand that was on the buttock or lower ribs up to the scapula. Simultaneously, glide the other hand down to the buttock or lower ribs.

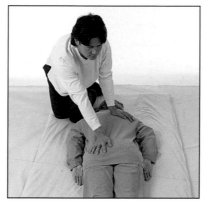

5. Now move the trailing knee over the receiver's head to rest next to the leading knee.

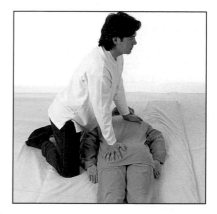

6. Move the leading knee adjacent to the receiver's waist or hips and make any necessary adjustments to your position for your comfort.

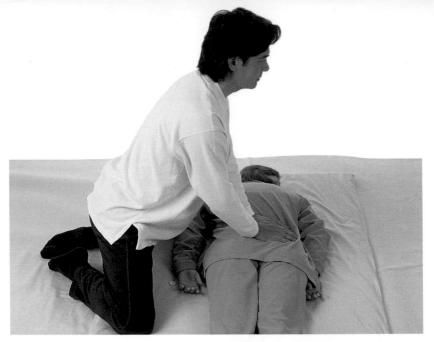

Rocking

K neel at right angles to your receiver and place both hands on her torso, on or near her waistline. If preferred, you can place one of your hands on her sacrum or hip. Rock her body from side to side. Attune to the rhythm that seems most natural for her, which you will recognize as the rhythm which is most effortless for you to maintain. Keep your arms, shoulders and spinal column loose and 'soft', allowing the rocking movement to come more from your belly and hips than from your arms. Being rocked is an inherently relaxing experience, as is evidenced by the way that babies are lulled when gently rocked, so this technique is useful to include at this stage if the receiver has not yet fully relaxed.

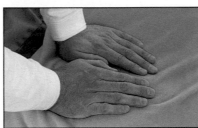

Mould your hands into the contours of your receiver's waistline, ensuring they are free of tension. 'Connect' rather than grab.

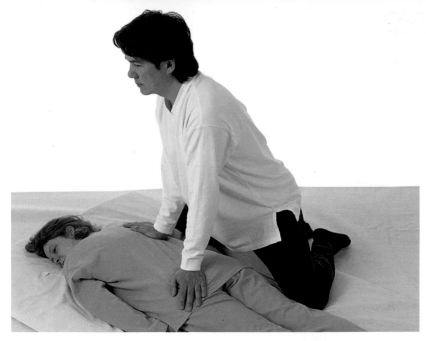

Diagonal stretch

P lace one hand on the near side of the receiver's upper back, with the heel of your hand close to the inside edge of the scapula (shoulder-blade) and the palm held flat against the lower half of the scapula. Your hand should be positioned no higher than this otherwise you will compress the receiver's neck. Place your other hand on the receiver's farside buttock so that your hands are positioned diagonally. Lean your hara forward towards the space between your hands and you will feel them tending to splay apart. Allow this splaying effect to take up the slack in the receiver's skin and flesh, thus giving her a diagonal stretch across her entire back. Keep your shoulders down, your belly relaxed and your head up. Move your hands to the opposite scapula and buttock and repeat. Readjust your kneeling position for optimum comfort.

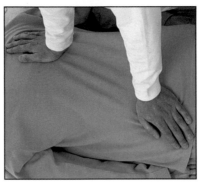

Place your upper hand partly below and partly over the receiver's shoulder-blade. Place your other hand on the opposite buttock. Lean forward, stretching the back diagonally.

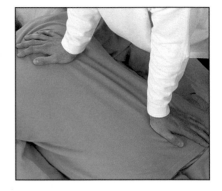

VARIATION

Follow the previous directions but place both hands on the same side of the body. This will 'open' one side of the back at a time in a longitudinal direction rather than diagonally.

NOTE IF KNEELING ON BOTH KNEES IS UNCOMFOR-TABLE, TRY HALF KNEELING WITH THE KNEE OF ONE LEG AND THE FOOT OF THE OTHER ON THE GROUND (SEE PAGE 40).

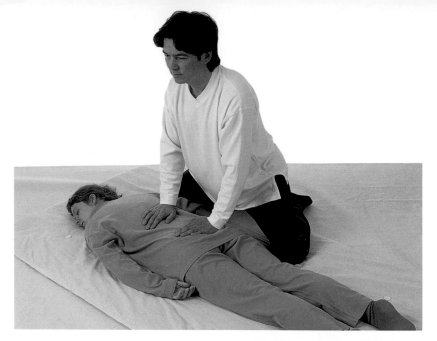

Sacral rub

Adopt whichever kneeling or squatting position suits you. Keep a support hand on the back of the receiver's torso or the back of her thigh. Place your other hand firmly on her sacrum (the bony area between the centre of her buttocks and her lower back). Rotate your hand as if polishing the bony sacrum with the skin covering it, so that the skin and the clothing over it is used like a cleaning rag, for 15–30 seconds. (*Do not* polish her skin or her clothing with the surface of your palm.) This technique generates a feeling of deep warmth which spreads from the sacrum throughout the entire body and is useful for people who tend to feel the cold. If your arms become tired, change hands every five seconds or so.

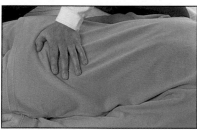

Circle the skin of the sacral area over the sacral bone.

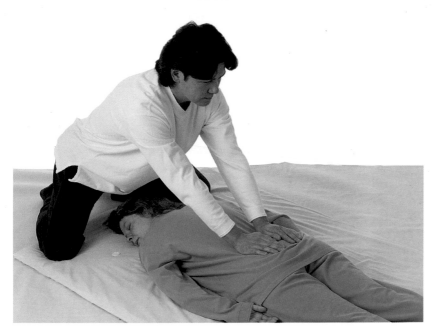

Retreating cat

Move from the side of the receiver's body to just beyond her head, facing her feet, using the first half of the procedure described in Moving to the Other Side (page 67). Glide both hands down her back until the heels of your hands rest into her buttocks. Lean your body weight forward for 1–2 seconds to stretch her buttocks away from her lower back, thus giving a gentle traction to her lower back. Now 'walk' your hands from her buttocks up to her shoulder, removing one hand after the other as if you were crawling backwards away from her lower back. If you like, you can 'walk' your hands into her upper arms. Repeat the Retreating Cat 3–4 times. Glide your hands gracefully into her buttocks; stretching them too suddenly or vigorously away from her lower back could weaken the ligaments of her lumbo-sacral joint and lower lumbar vertebrae.

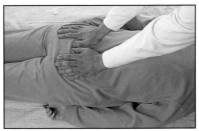

1. Make sure your hands are well on the buttocks to ensure a gentle traction to the lower back.

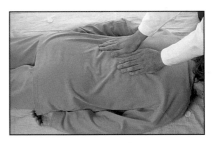

2. Walk your hands from the buttocks back up to the shoulders.

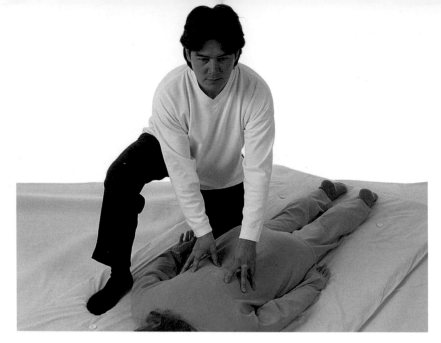

Thumbs down Bladder Channel on torso

A Ki channel known as the Bladder Channel begins in the depression slightly above the inner corner of the eye and runs over the head and down the back about 1^1/$_2$ thumb-widths either side of the vertebral column, all the way into the bony sacrum and down the leg to the foot. This line down the back is known as the inner line. Another branch called the outer line runs parallel to it at a distance of three thumb-widths from the vertebral column.

Locate the bony protuberances (the spinous processes) of the vertebral column. Adopt a wide kneeling, half kneeling or squatting position behind the receiver's head. Starting in her upper back, below the base of her neck, glide your thumbs either side of the spine to a position about 1^1/$_2$ thumb widths lateral to the vertebral column. Lean in with your thumbs so that the angle of pressure is at right angles to the contour of

her back. Sink your thumbs in using your body weight, not strength. Check with the receiver that you are not causing her any degree of pain. Withdraw your thumbs and glide them adjacent to the space between the next knobbly spinous processes. Continue working down the receiver's back in this manner until you reach a stage where it is no longer possible for you to keep your hara in line with the neck of the tsubo that you are working on.

To maintain the correct angle of entry into the tsubos of the Bladder Channel, change your position by moving away from the receiver's head and adopting a half-kneeling position by her side, facing towards her head. Work down her lower thoracic region into the lumbar area, if necessary shuffling your position slightly as you move down to make yourself comfortable. As you work towards and onto the sacrum (buttock area) you may

prefer to turn and face the receiver's feet in order to ensure the correct angle of entry into the tsubo.

Go back to the head of the receiver's body, facing her feet, trying not to take your hands off her body as you do so. Repeat, but this time work three thumb-widths from the midline vertebral column.

Where the Bladder Channel runs along the spine it has points which relate to different organs and functions of the body. Experienced practitioners may focus on these points (tsubos) in order to alleviate specific problems, but at foundation course level it is sufficient for you to know that by working down the Bladder Channel in a generalized way as described in this technique you will be encouraging greater harmony between all the receiver's bodily functions.

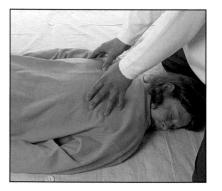

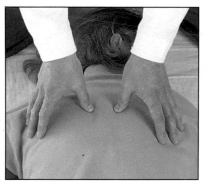

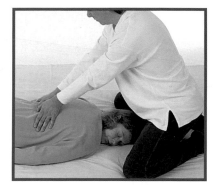

Position your thumbs so that the angle of pressure is at right angles to the contour of the back.

The correct position of the thumbs, adjacent to the space between the spinous processes.

The thumbs are too far down the receiver's back in relation to the giver's position, so that the giver's hara is no longer aligned with the neck of the tsubo.

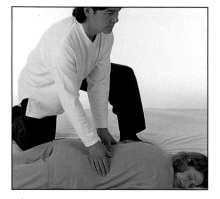

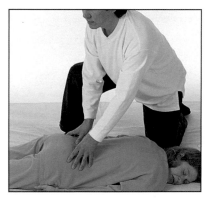

1. In half kneeling, facing towards her head, work down the lower thoracic area of the Bladder Channel, either side of the spine.

2. In half kneeling, work on the lower lumbar and sacrum area, facing towards the receiver's feet if you prefer.

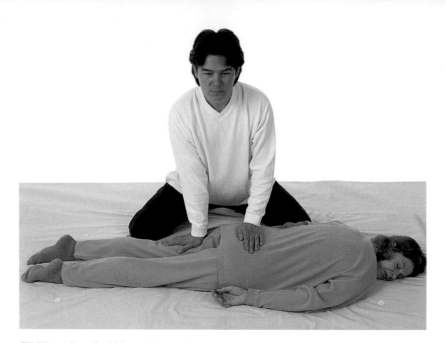

4.9

Palm/forearm down back of legs

Kneel or half kneel beside the receiver with one knee or foot adjacent to her hip and the other adjacent to her knee or lower leg. Place your support hand on her sacrum or nearside buttock and use the other hand to palm down the back of her thigh as far as the back of the knee. Do not lean pressure into the back of her knee, although you can make a light connection there with your palm.

Move your position closer to her feet so that your support hand now rests on her lower thigh. Palm down towards her heels. Do not lean excessive pressure into her calf, as this is often a very sensitive area.

Without breaking contact, move back up so that your knee is again adjacent to her hip. This time rest a hand or forearm against her buttock for support and use your other forearm to lean pressure into the back of her thigh. Do not look down, but feel your way.

Finally, move your position closer to her feet so that you can again rest a support hand on her lower thigh, and repeat palming your hand towards her heels.

The back of the legs relates predominantly to the Bladder Channel, so working this area immediately after using your thumbs down the Bladder Channel in the torso will give the receiver a better sense of 'connectedness' between her torso and her legs.

NOTE AVOID THE LEGS IF VARICOSE VEINS ARE PRESENT BECAUSE DIRECT PRESSURE ON VARICOSE VEINS IS EXTREMELY PAINFUL AND MAY CAUSE THEM DAMAGE.

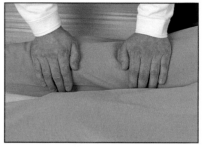

1. Rest your support hand on the lower thigh as your other hand palms down towards the feet.

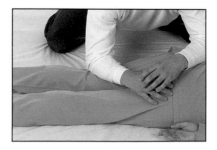

2. Rest your forearm against the receiver's buttock for support and use your other forearm to lean pressure into the back of her thigh.

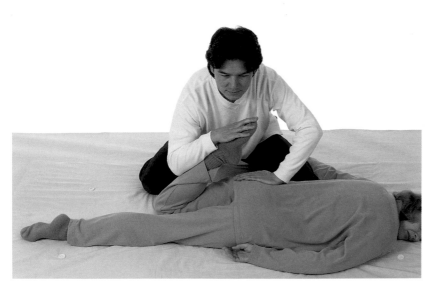

Heel to buttock

With one knee adjacent to the receiver's hip and the other approximately adjacent to her knee, place your support hand on her buttock and your other hand under her instep. Keeping your chest within 30cm (12 inches) of her foot, bring her heel towards her buttock, at the same time using your support hand to stretch her buttock away from her lower back. The movement should be performed in a slightly circular rather than linear manner so that you bring the heel towards the buttock along a semi-circular path and draw it back in a similar fashion.

If the receiver's heel does not easily reach her buttock, recognize the point of resistance and do not force the stretch. If the receiver is so flexible that she feels no stretch in the thigh muscles with this technique, you can increase the stretch by raising her thigh upon your own before leaning her heel towards her buttock.

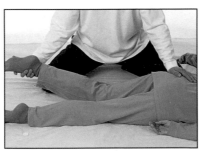

1. The starting position: the support hand is on the buttock and the other hand is under the instep.

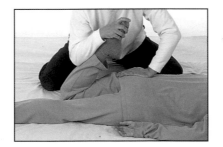

2. Bring her heel towards her buttock, simultaneously stretching her buttock away from her lower back with your support hand.

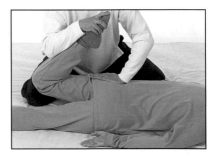

3. To increase the stretch for flexible recipients, raise her knee onto your thigh prior to applying the stretch.

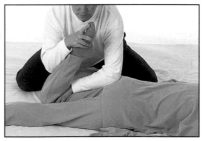

VARIATION
This variation gives less stretch to the front of the thigh but 'opens' the front of the knee joint by way of slight leverage. Because your hand is sandwiched behind the knee, the front of the knee is stretched open a little.

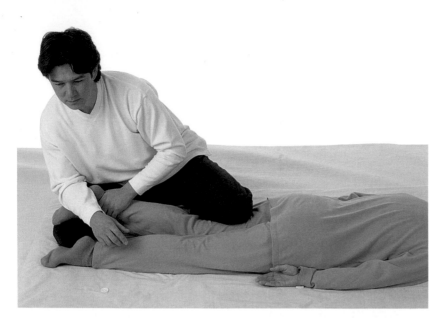

Forearms into soles

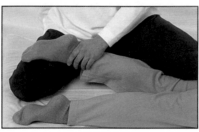

Make sure the receiver's instep moulds precisely into the contour of your thigh to give full support to her foot.

When you bring the receiver's leg down out of the Heel to Buttock technique, position your thigh so that her instep comes to rest upon it. The concave shape of her instep should fit precisely into the convex contour of your thigh, so that her foot is fully supported and not dangling in mid-air. Your other knee should rest on the back of her thigh, although if this is difficult you can rest it on the floor. Lean your forearm into the sole of her foot, keeping your wrist fully relaxed.

Because the soles of the feet are our main connecting points to the earth, leaning good solid pressure into them will give a sense of groundedness, particularly for those who are rather fuzzy-headed. Apart from that, this technique also feels very pleasant to receive. However, as some people have extremely sensitive feet, ask your receiver if she is actually enjoying it and if not, stop!

Moving to the other side

This sequence shows you how to get to the other side of the receiver's body smoothly and without breaking contact. Upon completion of this manoeuvre you will be in the correct position to repeat the entire leg sequence from 4.9 to 4.11 from the other side of the receiver.

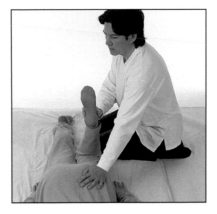

1. Bring her heel towards her buttock. Position your leading knee so that there is enough space between your knee and her nearside knee for you to place your trailing knee.

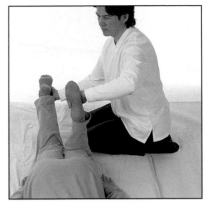

2. Adjust your hands so that the hand that was on the buttock now holds the nearside foot. Use your other hand to raise her other foot from the ground.

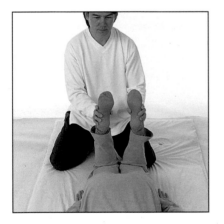

3. Now move your leading knee to the floor beyond her farside knee, leaving sufficient room for the trailing knee to be placed.

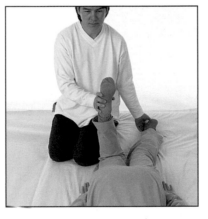

4. As you move your trailing knee towards your leading knee, lower her far side foot to the ground.

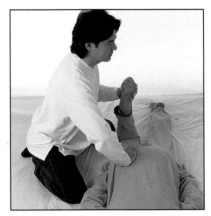

5. Now position your hands and adjust your leg position as if to perform the Heel to Buttock stretch on this side.

REPEAT THE TECHNIQUES 4.9 TO 4.11 FROM THE OTHER SIDE OF THE RECEIVER

SUPINE SEQUENCE

When giving shiatsu in this position, ask your receiver if she would like a pillow under her head. If she is very round-shouldered her chin will protrude upwards, constricting the back of her neck and overstretching the front, and she will be more comfortable with a block of 2.5–5cm (1–2in) thickness beneath her head. A book or a very stiff cushion will suffice. Before you begin, try to reach an attunement with the receiver by spending about a minute kneeling by her with one hand resting on her hara and your other hand holding her wrist or hand, as shown here.

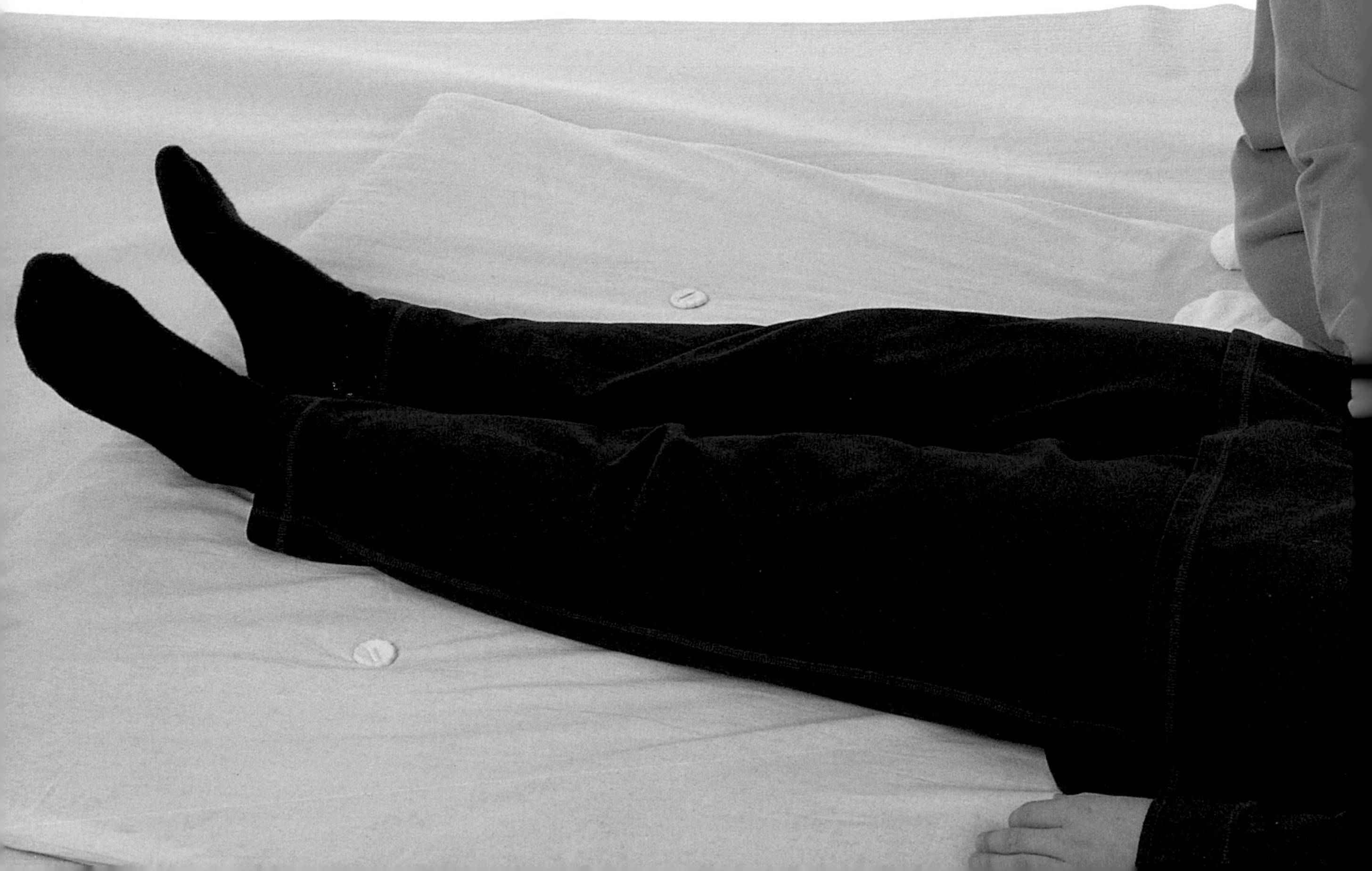

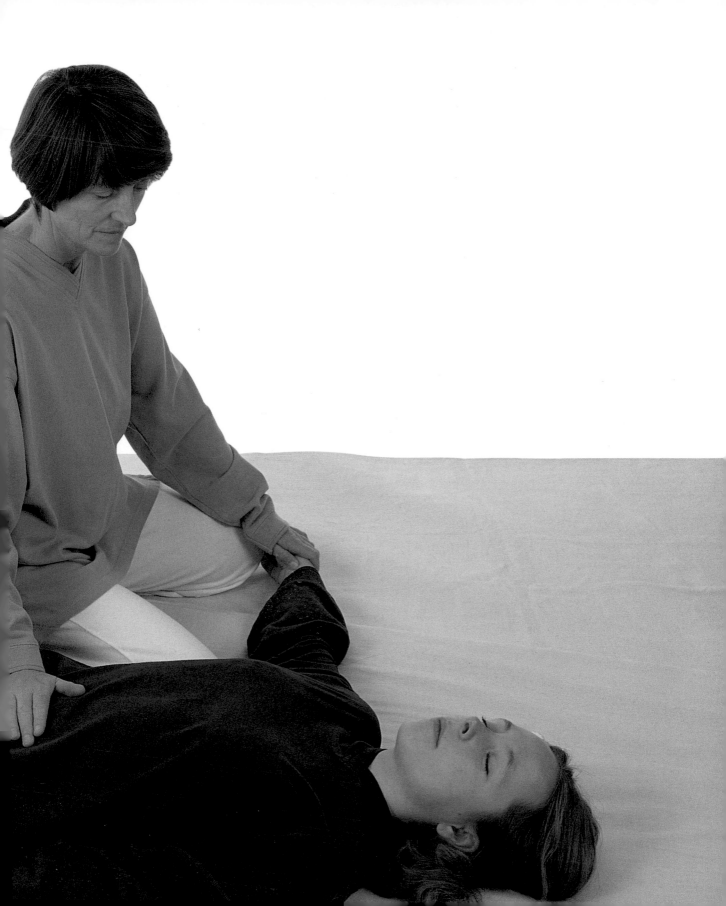

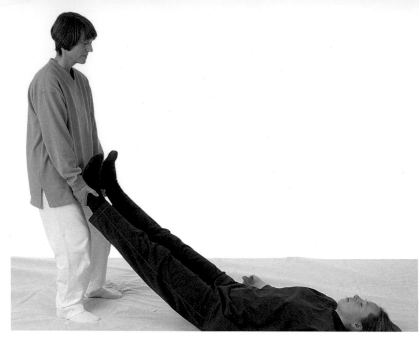

Pulling heels

T his technique gently stretches the recipient's spine. Stand at the receiver's feet, facing towards her head. Place your hands under her heels and pick up her feet. Ensure her heels are lifted high enough for her lower back to flatten against the floor, otherwise you may exaggerate your own lumbar curve. Do not clutch her ankles; hold onto the bony part of her heels. Adopt a stance with your knees slightly bent and your feet slightly apart and hold her feet close to your belly or chest.

If the receiver has hyper-extended knee joints (knees which seem to bend the other way slightly when the leg is meant to be straight) as well as heavy legs, avoid this technique.

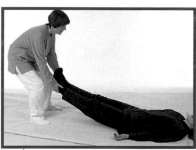

Here the heels are insufficiently raised, causing an exaggerated lumbar curve for the receiver when the giver leans back to pull the heels. This may result in back pain for the receiver.

The correct hand position, holding the bony part of the heels rather than clutching the ankles.

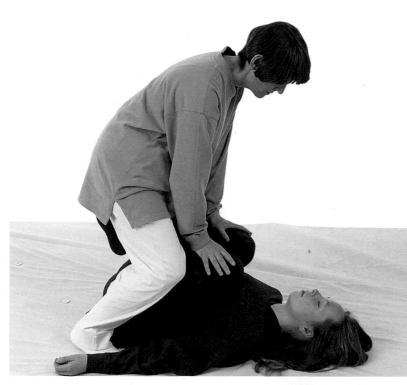

Double knee to chest

Still holding the receiver's heels, walk forwards as you raise her heels level with your chest. You may want to rest her heels on your chest for a moment as you put your hands behind her knees. Allow her knees to bend as you walk your feet adjacent to her hips, using the inside surface of your knees or lower legs to support and control her legs. Gently lean some of your weight through your hands straight down onto her legs, allowing her knees to spread to avoid pressure on her aorta (the main blood vessel from the heart). This will give a subtle 'opening' stretch to her lower back and buttocks and will help decongest her colon.

To move out of this technique, see right.

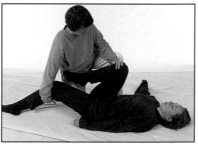

Half-kneel to the side of one of the receiver's hips and lower her legs to the ground, one at a time. Ensure you support the back of her knee as you do so. This option works better on the smaller, lighter receiver.

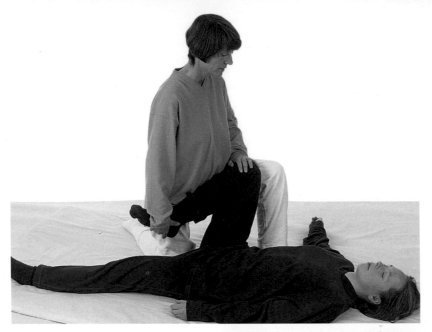

Hip circling

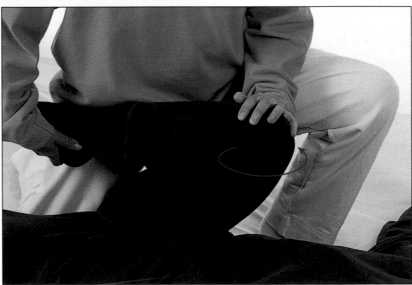

There are several versions of Hip Circling. The three most popular options are given here. All involve bending one of the receiver's legs towards her chest and drawing outward circles in the air with her knee. The Hip Circling technique gently mobilizes the hip joints and increases circulation to the hips and sacrum.

Hip Circling illustrates how truly relaxed your receiver is because unless she is fully at ease she will hold tension in her leg throughout the movement, often doing the movement herself instead of allowing you to do it. If this is the case Version B should work better because the extra support will make it easier for her to let go. Give her plenty of time and encouragement so that she feels able to 'give' her leg to you.

VERSION A

Adopt the half-kneeling position to one side of the receiver's hip. Hold her knee with one hand and her heel with the other. Bend her knee towards her chest. Draw outward circles in the air with her leg, exploring the natural range of movement in her hip joint. This method allows for the maximum circumference of hip rotation. Alternatively, you can keep your leg in contact with her moving leg instead,

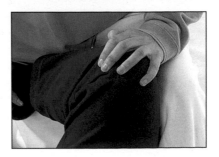

which slightly restricts the range of movement but adds a greater sense of 'connection'.

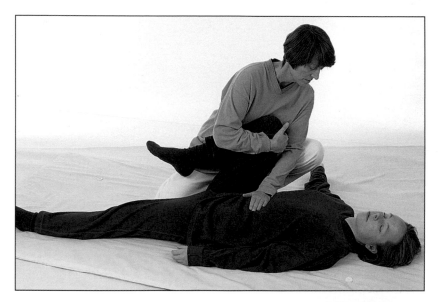

VERSION B

Adopt the wide kneeling position. Place one hand on the receiver's belly. Hold her knee with your other hand, hugging her folded leg between your chest and forearm. Rotate her hip joint by circling your torso from your hara, thereby circling her leg. This method does not allow full circumference of hip rotation, but gives a much greater sense of nurturing and connection.

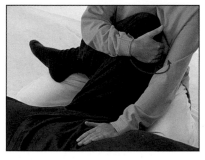

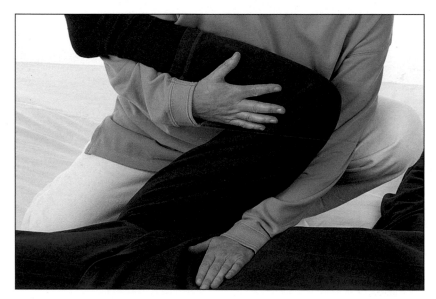

VERSION C

This version of Hip Circling is the same as Version B except that the receiver's lower leg is cradled by your forearm. Some receivers may find this version rather too intimate and consequently fail to relax into it. This technique may also be done in the squat kneeling position if you find it more comfortable.

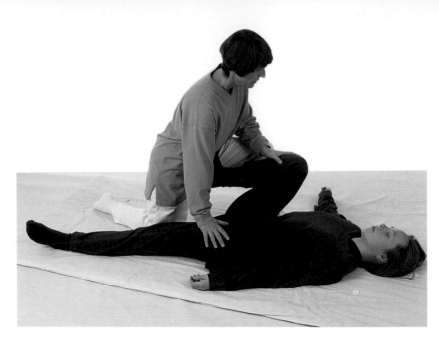

Single knee to chest

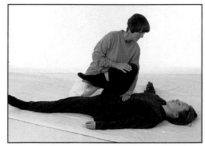

Either version of Hip Circling can be progressed into the Single Knee to Chest technique by simply leaning some of your weight towards the receiver's chest, keeping one hand on either her belly, or the straight leg. This can be helpful if that leg has a tendency to lift up as you lean some of your weight on to the bent leg. On some people the knee will more naturally move to the side of their torso; on others, the knee will move directly towards the chest. Go with her natural direction. The technique will stretch the lower back and buttocks and help to decongest the colon.

Do this technique slowly so that you go no further than is comfortable for the receiver. If she does begin to feel discomfort her back and neck may stiffen, causing her chin to protrude

This variation is a logical progression from Version B of Hip Circling. Adopt wide kneeling or squat kneeling (see pages 40–41) and keep one hand on the receiver's belly as you apply gentle pressure on to the bent knee.

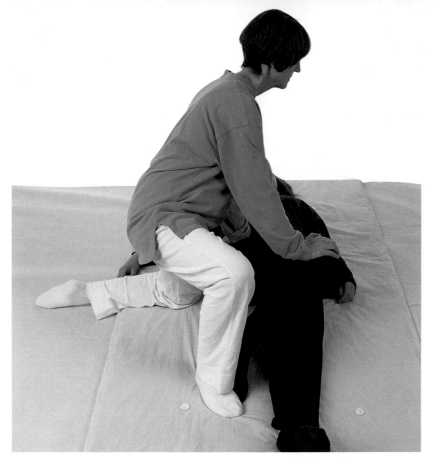

Stretch outside of thigh

This stretch 'opens' the channel relating to the Gall Bladder. Place the receiver's foot on the floor next to the knee of her straight leg, with her knee pointing towards the ceiling. Place one hand on her knee and your other hand firmly on her hip to anchor it. Place your foot or knee (depending on whether you are half kneeling or squat kneeling) against her foot to prevent it from slipping. Then give a slow stretch to the lateral side of her thigh by leaning her knee away from you. Sometimes it works better if the foot of the receiver's bent leg is placed across her straight leg, with her foot against the outside of her straight leg knee.

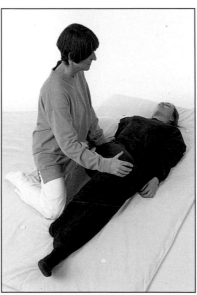

In the squat kneeling position, the giver's knee anchors the receiver's foot to prevent it sliding away.

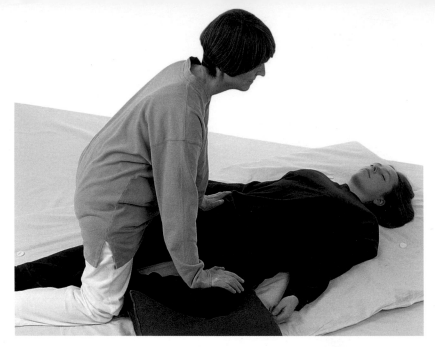

Opening inside leg and pelvis

Keeping the receiver's leg in the same starting position as the previous technique, adjust your legs to the opposite half-kneeling position. Place a cushion or two on the floor where her knee will rest when you lower her knee outwards towards the ground. As you lower her knee, switch your hand position so that the hand that was on the hip now supports the knee and the hand that was on the knee moves to anchor the upper thigh/hip of the far side leg. Gently 'open' her pelvis and inner thigh muscles by leaning the knee gently into the supporting cushions. Do not look down, but let your hara relax down. You may need more cushions, depending on the receiver's flexibility. If you do not have cushions nearby, allow her knee to be supported by your lower leg or inner ankle.

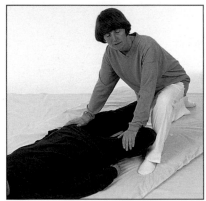

If no cushion is available, the receiver's knee can be supported by the giver's lower leg.

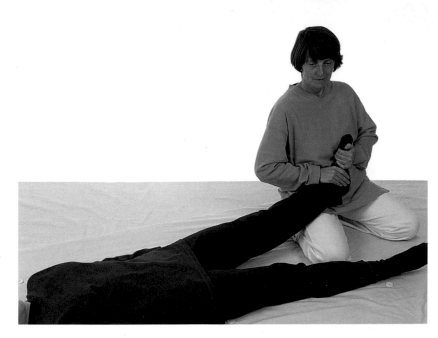

Foot to hara

Support the receiver's leg as you straighten it and position yourself in wide kneeling so that the outside edge of her foot rests squarely in your hara, embraced by your two hands. Lean your hara into her foot and circle her foot using your whole body. If the receiver has hyperextended knees (knees that bend the wrong way slightly) or experiences discomfort in her knee during this technique, use one hand or some cushions to support the back of her knee, thus keeping her knee 'unlocked'.

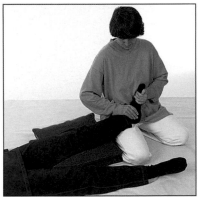

Provide support beneath the knee by means of a cushion if the receiver has hyperextended knees or is experiencing discomfort.

REPEAT TECHNIQUES 3 TO 7 ON THE OTHER LEG, TRYING NOT TO BREAK CONTACT AS YOU TAKE YOUR TIME MOVING ACROSS.

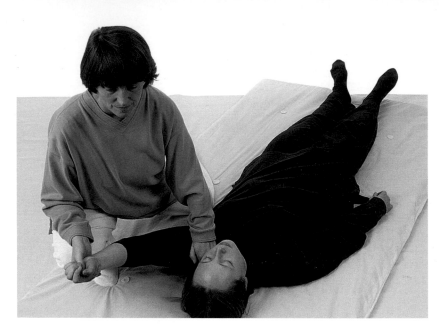

Arm circling and palming down arm

Move from the receiver's foot to her arm slowly and carefully, trying to maintain hand-to-body contact throughout. Cup one hand on the receiver's upper chest and shoulder and the other hand close by on her upper arm. Lean down with fairly firm supportive pressure for about 10 seconds. This will encourage her shoulder joint to 'let go'. Now move your hand from her upper arm to her wrist, with your thumb held against the palm of her hand. Take a step back with your outside leg and bring her hand to your own shoulder, simultaneously adjusting the hand which is on her shoulder to ensure sufficient purchase to stretch her shoulder. Take a big step forward with your outside leg to stretch her arm beyond her head. Step forwards and backwards two or three times to rotate the shoulder joint. The receiver's arm should be taken forward through a vertical arc and brought back through a horizontal arc close to the floor. You should maintain some traction to the shoulder joint throughout, particularly when you take the arm upwards and forwards.

Now place her arm on the floor at right angles to her torso. Palm down her arm towards her wrist, keeping one foot on her palm if you can remain comfortable like that as this will create an extra connection. If not, place your foot somewhere on the ground that feels more comfortable. Try to keep your other leg in contact with the side of her body to give maximum connection. If her arms are very long in relation to your size, place her arm closer to her body and, if necessary, sacrifice the connection of your leg against her torso.

Arm Circling mobilizes the shoulder joint, increasing the circulation of Ki and blood to the shoulder and chest area.

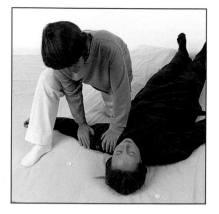

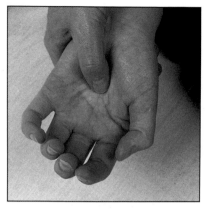

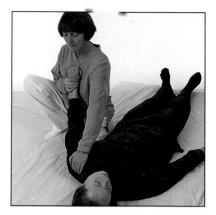

1. *Place one hand on the receiver's upper chest and shoulder and the other hand on her upper arm.*

2. *Move your hand from her upper arm to her wrist and place your thumb against her palm.*

3. *Stepping back with your outside leg results in a stretch to the recipient's trapezius muscle.*

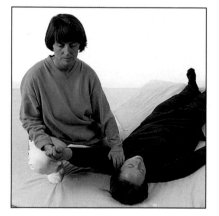

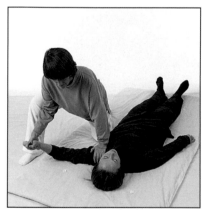

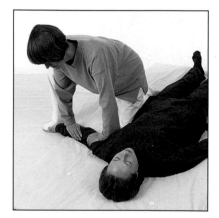

4. *A big step forwards allows you to stretch the receiver's arm up beyond her head.*

5. *Repeat Arm Circling two or three times, bringing the arm back in a horizontal arc close to the ground.*

6. *Lay the receiver's arm on the ground at right angles to her torso and palm down her arm towards her wrist.*

NOTE ROTATE THE RECEIVER'S ARM OVERHEAD ONLY AS FAR AS SHE CAN GO BEFORE HER SHOULDER TIGHTENS UP – DO NOT TAKE THE ARM TO THE FLOOR IF IT WILL NOT EASILY GO THERE. THIS IS LIKELY TO BE THE CASE IF YOUR RECEIVER IS ROUND-SHOULDERED.

Moving to the other side via the head

There are several ways to get from one side of the receiver's body to the other without taking both your hands off her body. The method shown here works particularly well if you are taller than the receiver. If you are shorter, just take a few extra shuffles with your knees as you go.

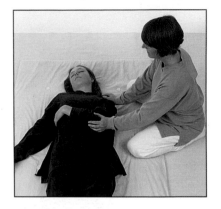

1. Kneeling with your knees well spread, place the receiver's forearm across her lower ribs, holding her elbow and shoulder.

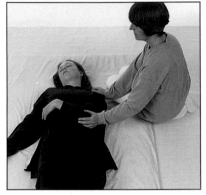

2. Make sure there is space between your leading knee and her shoulder. Place your trailing knee next to your leading knee.

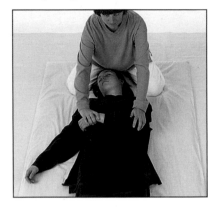

3. Move your leading knee to the floor on the other side of her head, making sure you leave space between your knee and her head. Simultaneously move your hand from her shoulder to her wrist.

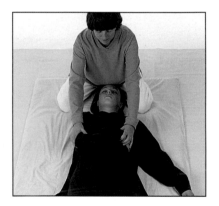

4. Place her arm back on the floor and bring her other forearm across her lower ribs.

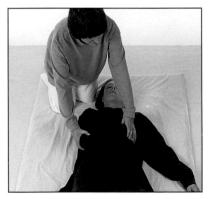

5. Place your trailing knee between her head and your leading knee.

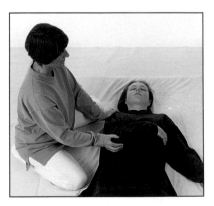

6. Move your leading knee near to her hip, at the same time moving your hand from her wrist to her shoulder.

REPEAT ARM CIRCLING AND PALMING DOWN ARM FROM THE OTHER SIDE ON THE ARM YOU ARE NOW HOLDING.

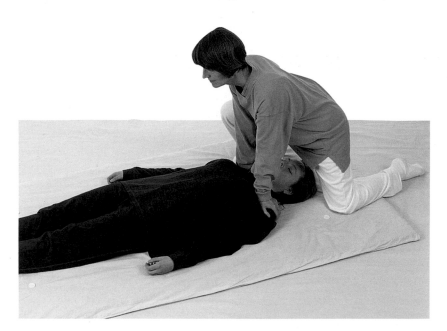

Shoulder press

Position yourself at the receiver's head, looking towards her feet. Check to see if she has round shoulders. If so, her shoulders will not lie flat upon the ground and her chin will project upwards. If this is the case, or if she has neck pain, follow the variation shown right. Otherwise proceed as follows: cup your hands over her shoulders, fingers to the rear. The heels of your hands should be on the upper chest muscles (pectoralis minor), in the hollow just below her clavicle (collarbone). Lean your hara forward so that your weight falls through your hands, 'opening' the receiver's upper chest. Be careful to keep your groin well away from her face. and tuck away any loose, dangling clothing to prevent it contacting her head.

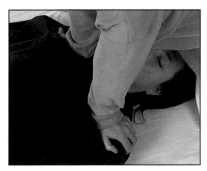

The heel of your hand should rest in the hollow just below the collarbone and your fingers should be to the rear.

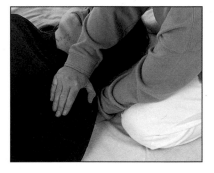

VARIATION

For those receivers who have round shoulders or neck pain or who are frail, place one hand underneath the shoulder to support it and place the other hand on the upper chest and shoulder, thereby sandwiching the shoulder between your hands. Lean through your upper hand. Repeat on the other shoulder.

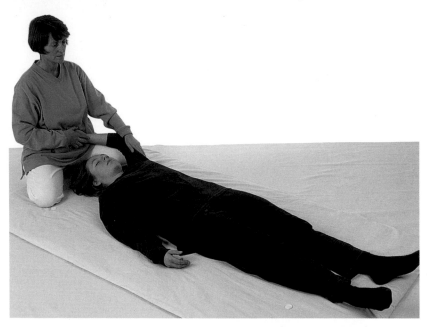

5.10

Hand to hara

This technique calms the Heart Channel and consequently calms the mind. Adopt the wide kneeling position. Bring one of the receiver's arms onto your thigh and hold the back of her hand against your hara. If you have her right hand in your hara, hold it with your left hand and vice versa. Rest your other hand on her armpit or upper arm, then slowly lean gentle pressure through your hand along her arm towards her elbow. Alternatively, a mild squeezing or stroking action can be applied. Sometimes it works better to lean your forearm in rather than use your hand.

To complete the technique, use two or three fingers of your other hand to apply gentle pressure to the anterior surface of the receiver's wrist, in line with her fifth finger. Repeat on her other arm. Replace her arm on the ground by her side to conclude.

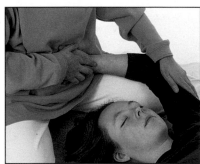

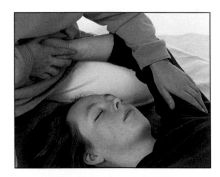

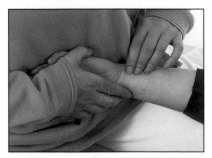

1. Support the receiver's arm on your thigh and hold her hand against your hara.

2. Gently lean through your hand along the receiver's upper arm and forearm.

3. Finally, use two or three fingers to apply gentle pressure to the anterior surface of her wrist, in line with her fifth finger.

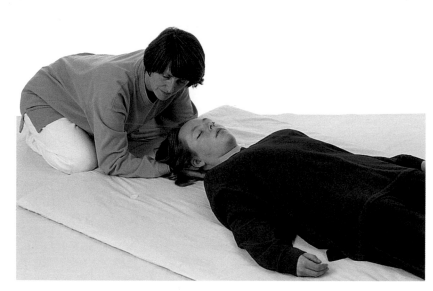

Fingertips into suboccipital area

Cradle the receiver's head in your hands and rest the back of your hands on the floor. Move your knees back far enough to rest your elbows on the floor and to allow your back, hara and chest to remain open and relaxed. Rest your fingertips into the area of the receiver's neck closest to the back of her skull (the occiput). By lightly flexing your wrists you can tilt her head back a little, allowing greater depth of contact with your fingertips.

To conclude this technique, and the supine sequence, gently withdraw your hands via the back of her head extremely slowly, thus giving a very mild lengthening effect to the back of her neck.

VARIATION
Some practitioners find it more comfortable to be positioned closer, sitting up with the receiver's head resting on their knees. Others find that this method closes the hara too much. Try both positions to see which suits you best.

NOTE A FULL SERIES OF NECK TECHNIQUES IS TAUGHT DURING A LATER STAGE OF TRAINING, BEYOND THE FOUNDATION COURSE, WHEN YOUR LEVEL OF TOUCH SENSITIVITY WILL BE MORE DEVELOPED.

SIDE SEQUENCE

Shiatsu in the side position has certain advantages over the prone or supine position as it enables full mobility of the shoulders, arms, hips and legs, plus greater movement of the torso. It is also useful for people with back problems and women in the later stages of pregnancy, who often find it difficult to relax fully in any position. To ensure the receiver is comfortable in the side position, place sufficient padding under the head and knee, as shown on page 98.

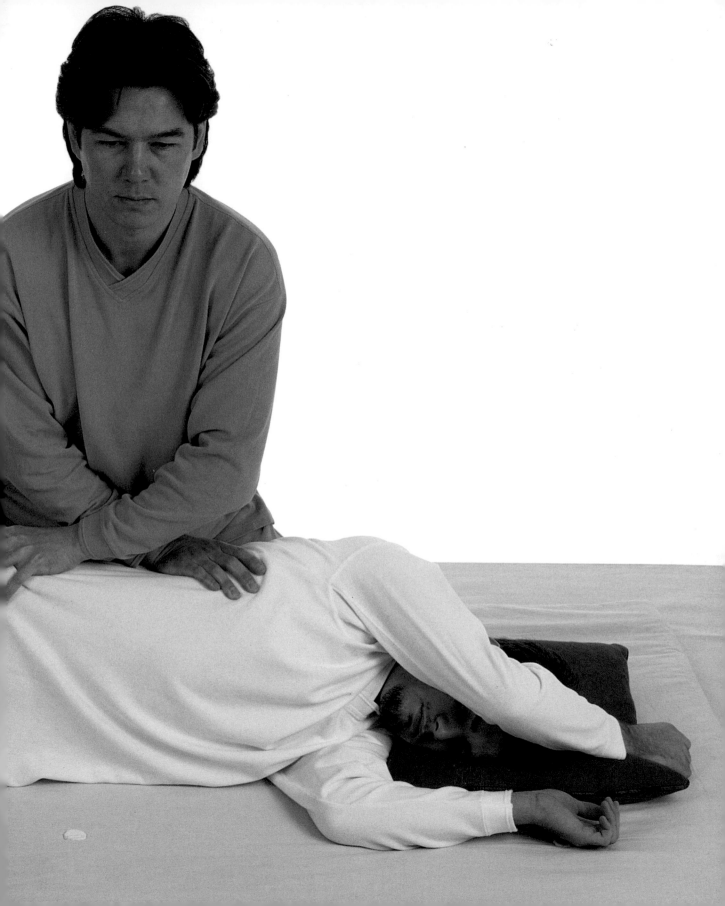

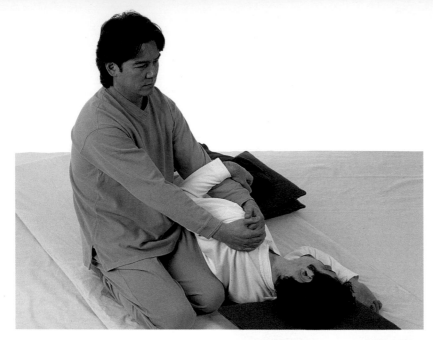

Trapezius stretch

Kneel in the seiza position next to the receiver, facing towards his head. Snuggle in close for maximum connection, but without pushing him off balance. Place his forearm over your forearm so that his arm does not drag on the floor. Clasping your hands around his shoulder, lean back, using your body weight to 'open' his neck (upper trapezius muscle). If his head comes away from the pillow you have leaned back far too strongly, so go more gently. Your hand position can be such that one hand overlaps the other, as shown here, or you can interlace your fingers. Do what you find most comfortable.

The Trapezius Stretch is a great antidote to the stress-induced tension that can so easily accumulate in the neck and shoulders.

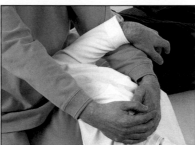

The receiver's forearm should be placed over your forearm to prevent his arm dragging on the floor.

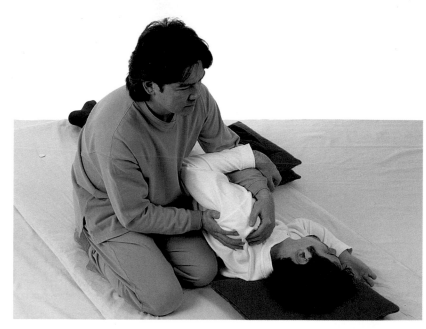

Shoulder girdle rotation

From the Trapezius Stretch, rotate the receiver's shoulder girdle in an up, back and down direction to encourage his chest to 'open'. Your whole body should be involved in the rotation, not just your arms. Alternate between the Trapezius Stretch and Shoulder Girdle Rotation for 1–2 minutes.

During this technique some receivers will involuntarily stiffen their shoulder as you try to rotate it. They will tend to relax more if you support the shoulder solidly between your hands. Receivers who are able to relax fully find this technique very pleasant.

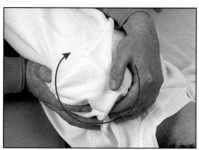

Correct technique: backward rotations encourage the chest to 'open'.

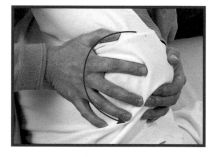

Incorrect technique: forward rotations encourage the chest to 'close'.

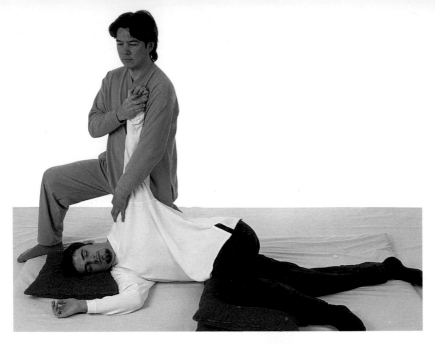

Vertical arm stretch

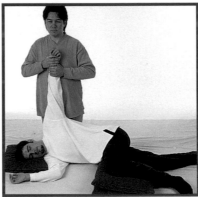

From Shoulder Girdle Rotation, remove your hand from behind the receiver's shoulder and clasp his hand. Leave your other hand on his shoulder and swivel up into half kneeling to face the same direction as he is facing. Sink down a little and embrace his arm, giving it as much contact as possible with your arm and torso. Straighten your posture. This will result in a traction of his shoulder girdle, shoulder, elbow and wrist joints.

Do not be tempted to hold his wrist with both hands, as this may cause undue strain to his wrist or elbow joints. Do not perform this technique from the high kneeling position because that will cause unnecessary stress to your lower back, especially if you have any history of weakness or injury to your back.

Incorrect technique: keeping both knees on the ground will cause stress to your lower back. Holding the receiver's wrist without supporting the rest of his arm will stress his shoulder, elbow and wrist joints and cause tension in your neck and shoulders.

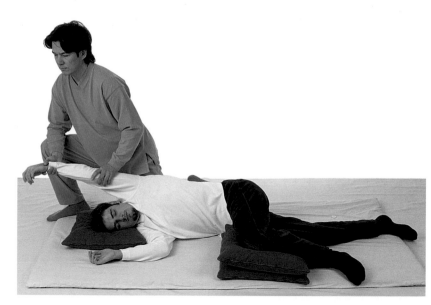

Lance stretch

From the Vertical Arm Stretch, change your grip to hold the receiver's wrist and circle his arm to a position where his arm is projecting beyond his head, so that there is a straight line between his upper hip, shoulder and hand. The hand that was holding his shoulder is now clasped around his upper arm. Rest your forearm upon your knee and lean away from the receiver's feet. This will 'open' the side of his ribs and torso. If his shoulder is stiff, stretch his arm slightly forward.

For this technique, it is best for your receiver to be wearing a long-sleeved garment as otherwise you could overstretch the skin of his upper arm. If he is wearing short sleeves, put a cloth between your hand and his arm.

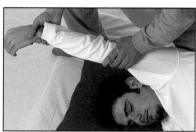

Hold the receiver's wrist and upper arm. Lean away from his feet to stretch his shoulder and 'open' the side of his ribs and torso.

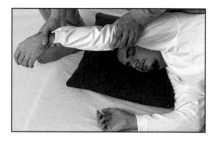

Stretch his arm slightly forward if his shoulder is stiff.

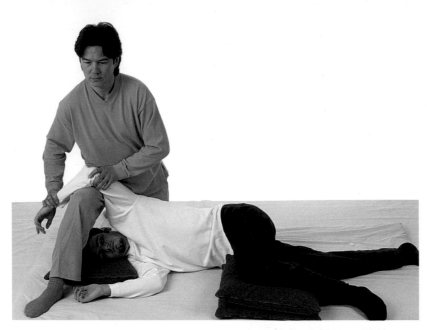

Bent arm lance stretch

Adjust your right foot, placing it well forward of the receiver's head. Allow his arm to bend over your thigh. Clasp his upper arm and hold his forearm. Now, just as in the straight arm Lance Stretch, lean away from his feet. This technique will 'open' the armpit area more than the straight arm Lance Stretch.

If you prefer, you can perform the technique in the squat kneeling position. This variation generally works better if your receiver has short arms or you have long legs.

The Bent Arm Lance Stretch helps to expand the ribcage and thus facilitates the ability to breathe more deeply.

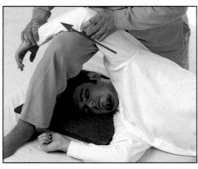

Place your foot well forward of the receiver's head so that your thigh can support his arm.

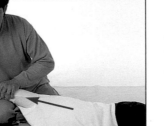

VARIATION
You can also perform this technique in a squat kneeling position. Experiment to see which method is most comfortable for you.

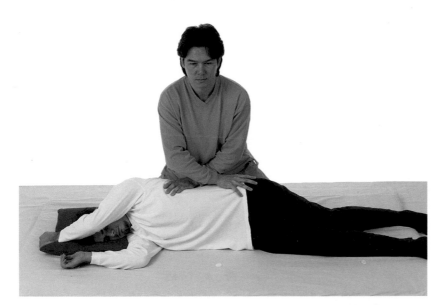

Side torso gall bladder stretch

Place the receiver's hand on the floor beyond his head or, if his shoulder joint lacks full mobility, in front of his chest. Kneel or half kneel behind him mid-way between his hip and shoulder. Place his upper leg to rest just behind his lower leg. This allows a greater stretch at the waist. If this is not comfortable for him, leave the leg where it was. Cross your arms and place one hand on his hip and the other hand on his lower ribs. Lean down and 'open' his waist area. Make sure you do not lean into his armpit or shoulder area as this will cause pain in his neck and shoulder.

This stretch gives the receiver a tremendous sense of 'freeing up' around the waist, lower back and belly. Using the forearms, as in the variation shown right, adds a more supportive, nurturing quality.

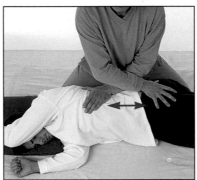

Leaning through crossed arms effectively 'opens' the waist area.

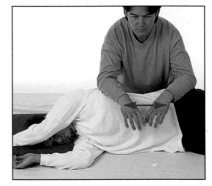

VARIATION
Try using your forearms instead of your hands. Again, avoid leaning too close to his armpit.

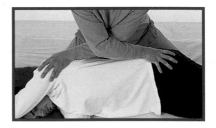

Incorrect technique: leaning into the receiver's armpit or shoulder will cause pain in his neck and shoulder.

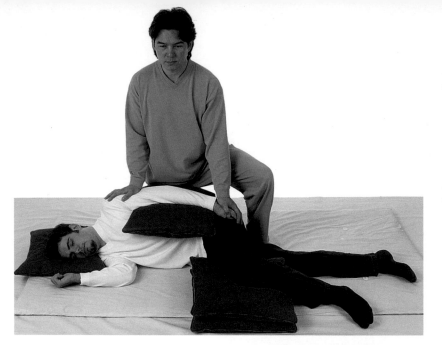

Arm to body stretch

Place the receiver's arm along his side with a cushion between his arm and his waist to avoid stressing his elbow joint. Lean your palms into varying areas along his arm and wrist. Do not lean too strongly into the corner of his shoulder as this may cause discomfort to his neck.

This technique is a good counter-movement to techniques 6.3, 6.4, 6.5 and 6.6. It also increases blood and Ki circulation throughout the arm and shoulder.

The forearm variation shown right adds a more warming, supportive quality. Take care not to push the receiver forward as you lean down.

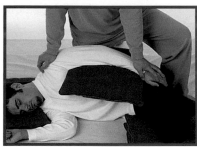

Incorrect technique: placing your hand too close to the corner of the receiver's shoulder may cause discomfort to his neck.

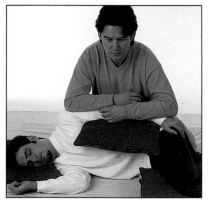

VARIATION

Try using your forearms instead of your hands. Again, avoid leaning too close to the receiver's armpit.

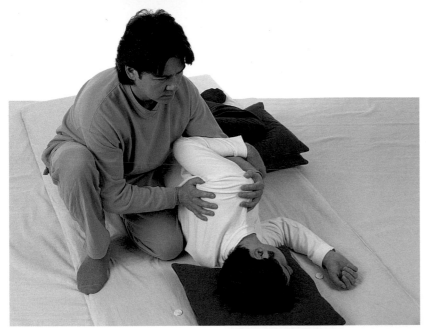

Shoulder girdle dispersing

Kneel or squat kneel next to the receiver, facing towards his head. Snuggle in close for maximum connection, but without pushing him off balance. Place his forearm over your forearm so that his arm does not drag on the floor. Support and anchor his shoulder with one hand while you vigorously circle the heel of your other hand into and around his scapula (shoulder-blade). Try to involve your torso in the movement as much as possible so that you minimize tension in your arm. However, your arm will still work quite hard in this technique. You can also try circling your hand slowly and deeply as a variation.

The purpose of this technique is to disperse tension in the muscles between the scapula and the vertebral column, so that the following technique (Sub-Scapula Loosening) can be achieved.

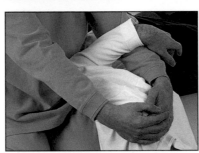

1. Place the receiver's forearm over your forearm to prevent his arm dragging on the floor.

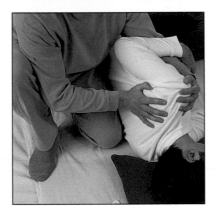

2. Circle the skin of the scapula area over the scapula bone.

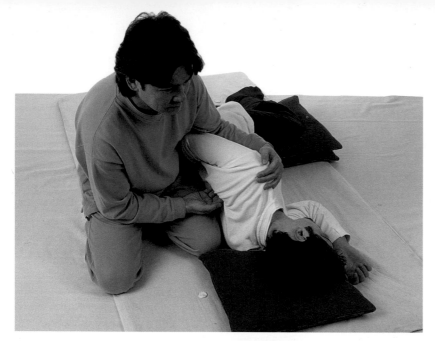

Sub-scapula loosening

Still supporting and anchoring his shoulder, place the receiver's hand behind his back. Place your fingertips under the inside edge of his scapula (shoulder blade) with your forearm resting on your thigh to anchor it, so that it becomes a fulcrum. Fold the receiver's scapula over your fingertips and lean away from his body, levering the scapula away from his ribcage a little. This looks extremely uncomfortable, but very few receivers feel any sensation at all during the technique, which is nicknamed 'the chicken wing'.

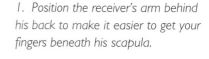

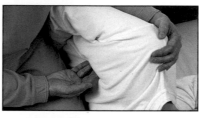

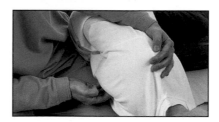

1. Position the receiver's arm behind his back to make it easier to get your fingers beneath his scapula.

2. Rest your forearm on your thigh to anchor it, thus reducing the need to tense your arm.

3. As you lean away the scapula is pulled away from the ribcage, releasing trapped Ki from that area.

NOTES YOU MAY FIND THAT YOU CANNOT GET YOUR FINGERS UNDER THE SCAPULA. IF SO, TRY VARIOUS ALTERATIONS TO THE RECEIVER'S ARM POSITION. IF YOU STILL CANNOT GET YOUR FINGERS IN, GIVE UP. SOME SCAPULAE ARE SIMPLY TOO SMALL OR TOO TIGHT AGAINST THE RIBS. WHEN ONE SCAPULA IS VERY MOBILE AND EASY TO GET UNDERNEATH AND THE OTHER IS TOO TIGHT, THIS OFTEN INDICATES A POSTURAL ANOMALY SUCH AS SCOLIOSIS (TWISTED SPINE). IF THE STIFF SCAPULA IS ON THE RIGHT IT CAN ALSO BE A SIGN OF A CONGESTED LIVER. PAIN UNDER THE LEFT SCAPULA MAY INDICATE CERTAIN STOMACH PROBLEMS SUCH AS STOMACH ULCER OR CHRONIC INDIGESTION.

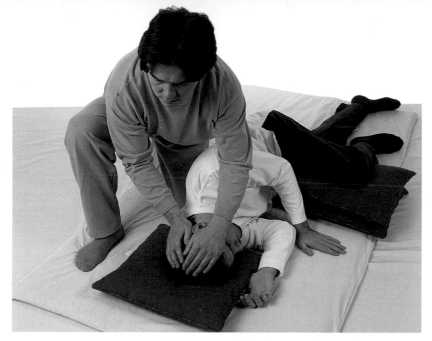

Head press

Come up into half kneeling or squat kneeling, facing towards the receiver's head. Place both palms on his head, being careful not to cover his ears. (You may wish to place a cloth between his head and your hands, especially if his hair is greasy.) Lean forward so that your weight drops through your hands – the pressure should obviously be gentle. Try to distribute your weight evenly throughout the palms of your hands rather than focusing it into the heels of your hands.

The channel relating to the gall bladder covers much of the side of the head and there are many points (tsubos) on this part of the channel which alleviate pain in the head, ears and eyes. This technique can therefore have a beneficial effect upon those symptoms. Note, however, that too much pressure will have the opposite effect.

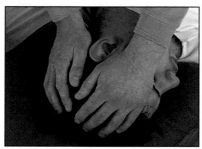

1. Place your hands on the receiver's head in such a way that you do not cover his ears.

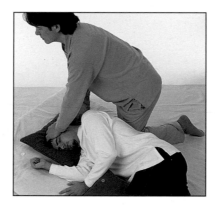

2. Lean forward so that you use your weight rather than your strength to apply pressure.

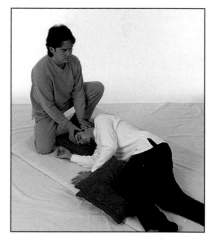

VARIATION
Adopt the same stances, but apply the technique from a position beyond the receiver's head, facing towards his feet.

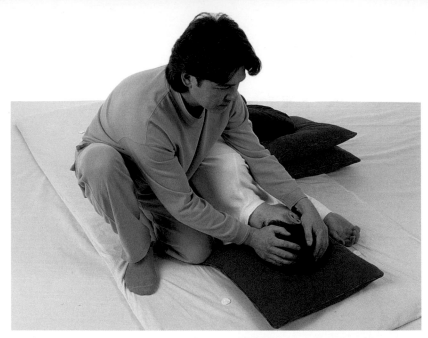

Occipital opening/neck release

Squat kneel beside the receiver. Snuggle in close for maximum connection, but without pushing him off balance. Place one hand on his forehead, without obstructing his eyes. Ideally, connect the front of his shoulder with your forearm (if it compromises your comfort, abandon this connection). Place the heel of your other hand against the nape of his neck and occiput. Explore this area with mild pressure.

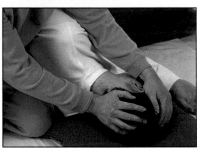

Palming the back of the head and neck can help relieve eye fatigue or a mild headache.

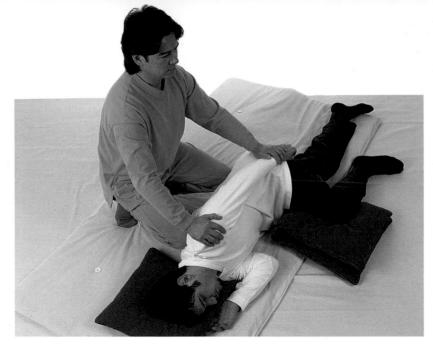

Knees into back

Squat behind the receiver with one hand on his shoulder and your other hand on his hip. Lean your knees against his back above his spinal column, upon the Bladder Channel found $1^1/_2$ thumb widths either side of the spine. Smoothly relocate your knees into various areas of his back between his buttocks and shoulder, keeping your knees above his spinal column. Avoid the tendency to round your back during this technique as you should keep your hara fully 'open' throughout.

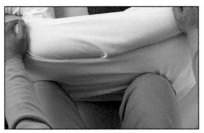

The correct knee position in relation to spinal column.

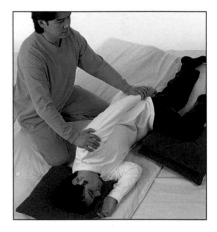

VARIATION

If you find this technique difficult using both knees together, place one knee on the floor so that you are in squat kneeling and use one knee only on the receiver's back.

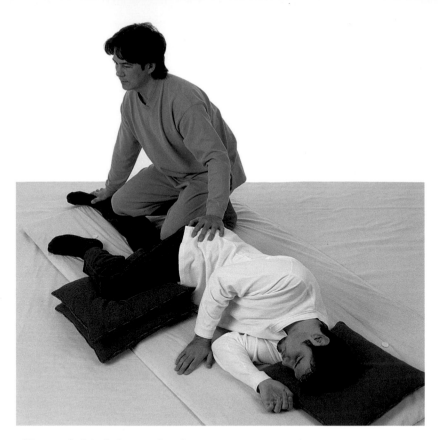

Kneeling on bottom leg

Squat behind the receiver's bottom leg with one hand on his hip and the other on his ankle or foot. Bring your knees onto his thigh and lower leg, controlling your knee pressure by taking the weight predominantly through your hands. With great care and sensitivity, 'walk' your knees into all accessible areas of his thigh and lower leg, avoiding his knee. Assuming the receiver finds this position comfortable, it should help to calm his mind.

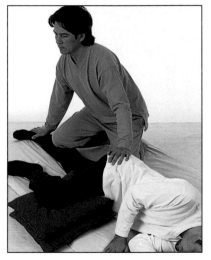

VARIATION
If you find this technique difficult using both knees together, place one knee on the floor so that you are in squat kneeling and use one knee only on the receiver's leg.

NOTE IF YOU FIND USING EVEN ONE KNEE TOO DIFFICULT, JUST PALM DOWN THE RECEIVER'S LEG.

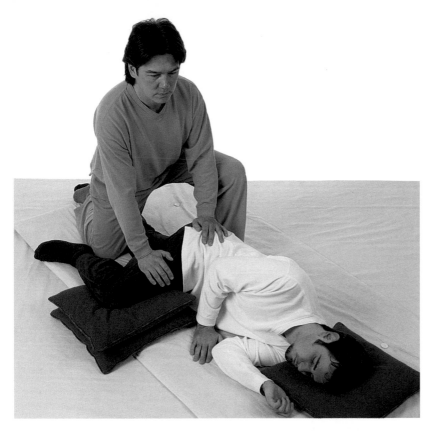

Palming the hip, thigh and lower leg

Adopt the half kneeling stance behind the receiver, straddling his bottom leg. Placing one of your thumbs on top of the other, locate the centre of his buttock. Slowly lean enough pressure into this point for him to feel a definite sensation (leaning too hard will cause sharp pain). Adjust your position so that you have a support hand on his hip and then lean your other palm progressively down the outside of his thigh towards his knee. Finish the technique by adopting a wide kneeling stance and use both hands to palm along his lower leg.

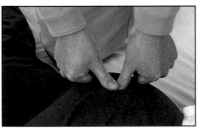

1. Place one thumb on top of the other in the centre of the receiver's buttock and lean pressure into this point. Don't lean in too strongly.

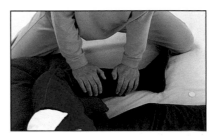

2. Adopt wide kneeling stance and use both hands to palm along the lower leg.

NOW GO BACK TO THE BEGINNING OF THE SIDE SEQUENCE AND REPEAT ALL THE TECHNIQUES ON THE RECEIVER'S OTHER SIDE.

SITTING SEQUENCE

For these techniques, ask your receiver to kneel in seiza or to sit with crossed legs. Many people find the latter more comfortable. They will find it easier to remain fully upright if they sit on a firm cushion or a foam block 5–7.5cm (2–3 inches) thick. In general, if your receiver is of similar height to you or smaller, you will find it easier to work on them if they kneel in seiza. If they are taller than you, it is usually easier to work on them if they sit cross-legged. Some people will not be comfortable in either position, in which case many of the following techniques can be done with them seated on a stool.

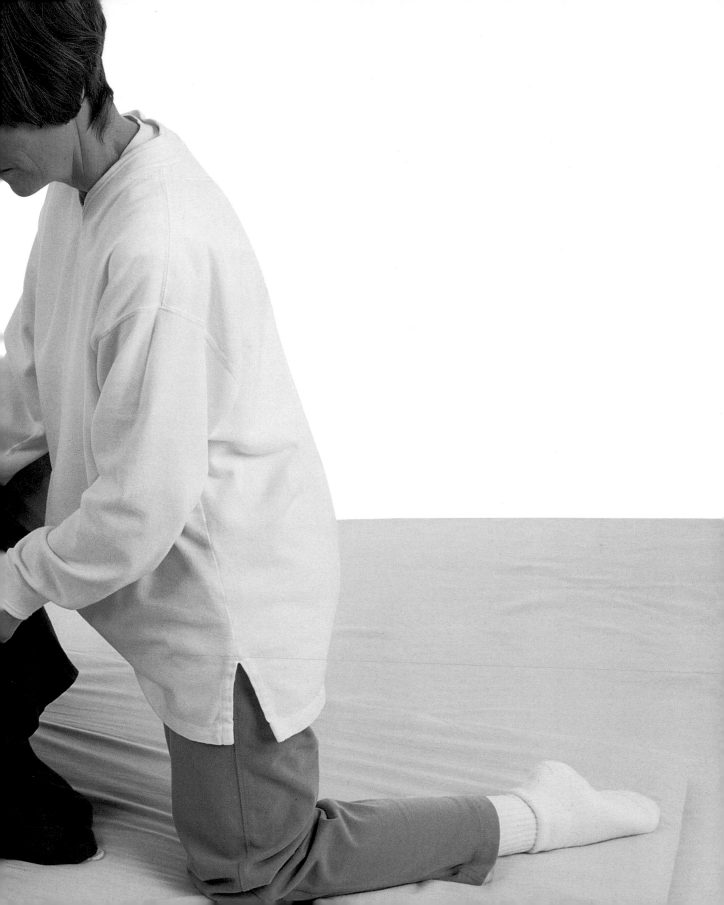

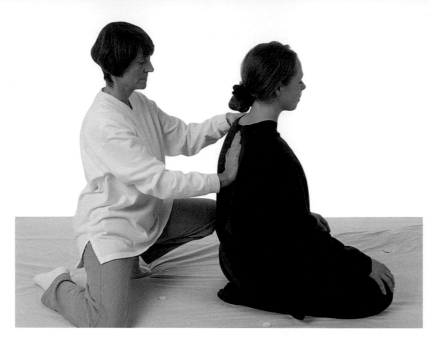

Palming down the spine

Kneel or squat kneel an arm's length behind the receiver. Place a support hand on her shoulder, close to the base of her neck (keep your fingers away from her throat). Leaning from your hara, use your other hand to palm down her back, either over her spine or to the side of the spine (the same side as the shoulder held by your support hand, as you will tend to twist her off balance if you palm the other side). Remember to keep your shoulders completely relaxed.

Repeat on the other side by placing your support hand on her other shoulder.

This is a good way to begin the sitting sequence because it enables you to feel easily whether or not the receiver is relaxed. It also encourages a better posture if she is slouching a little.

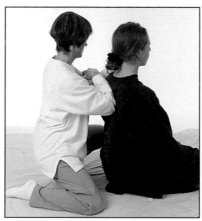

VARIATION
Position yourself closer to the receiver and use your forearm rather than your palm on her upper back. Move back and revert to using your palm on her lower back.

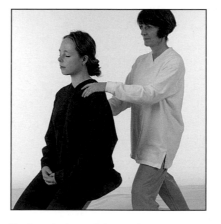

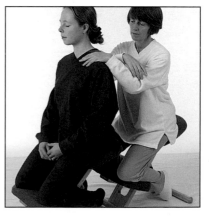

Both variations of this technique can be carried out with the receiver seated on a chair or stool while the giver stands or also sits on a stool.

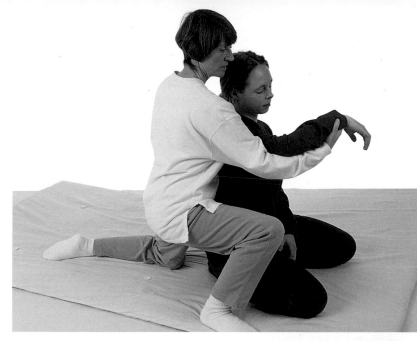

Arm circling

In half kneeling beside and slightly behind the receiver, place your support hand over her shoulder. If you are able to find an indentation behind her shoulder, this is a good place to put your thumb. This indentation is a point called Small Intestine 10.

Now cradle her arm in yours and rotate her arm backwards in a way that resembles the arm movement of swimming backstroke. Make sure you pass her arm well in front of her torso, which reflects a natural movement for her shoulder joint. Repeat on the other arm.

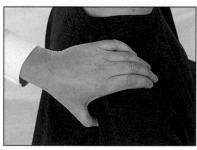

Place your support hand on the receiver's shoulder with your thumb in the indentation behind the shoulder.

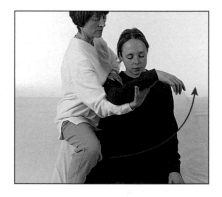

Correct technique: the arm is passed well in front of the torso, reflecting the natural movement of the shoulder.

NOTE: THIS TECHNIQUE CAN EASILY BE APPLIED WITH THE RECEIVER SEATED ON A STOOL AND THE GIVER STANDING RATHER THAN KNEELING. IF THE RECEIVER HAS LONG ARMS, YOU MAY NEED TO STEP FORWARDS AND THEN BACK AGAIN WITH YOUR OUTSIDE FOOT AS YOU CIRCLE HER ARM.

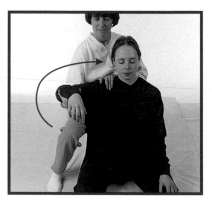

Incorrect technique: the receiver's arm is not passed sufficiently across the front of her torso.

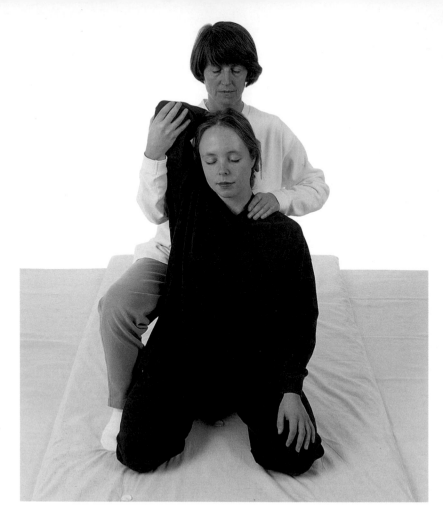

Single arm overhead stretch

Progressing directly from Arm Circling, keep the same arm cradled in your arm and place your support hand on the receiver's other shoulder, close to the base of her neck. Bring her arm over her head, thus giving her inner arm and armpit a mild 'opening' stretch. Repeat on the other arm.

It is easy to cause damage to the shoulder if this technique is applied with too much zeal, so, as usual, never force; simply 'take up the slack'.

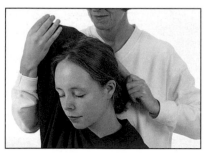

VARIATION

A minor variation to this technique is to place one hand on the receiver's elbow and hold her hand with the other.

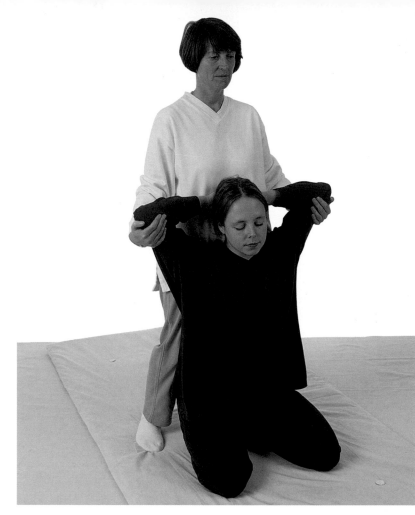

Armpit/chest stretch

With the receiver clasping her hands behind her neck, stand behind her and hold her elbows. Ask her to allow her head to relax forwards naturally and encourage her to relax and release her whole upper body as you gently ease her elbows back. Keep your knees and thighs in contact with her back. Synchronize the opening of her chest with the rhythm of her exhalations as this will make her feel she is in control of the stretch.

This technique helps to release stiffness in the muscles of the upper chest, expands the ribs and gently stretches the diaphragm. It therefore helps to improve breathing and posture. It also 'opens' the Heart Channel, which runs along the inner surface of the arm from the armpit to the fifth finger. The Heart Channel has a direct relationship with the mental focus, so if your receiver is a little sleepy this technique will perk her up. Conversely, if she is slightly agitated it may help to calm her.

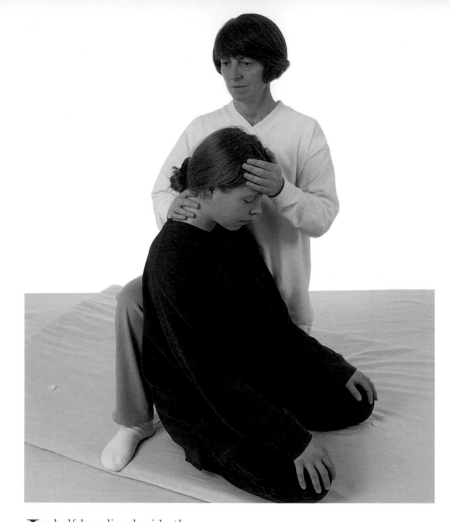

Forward neck stretch

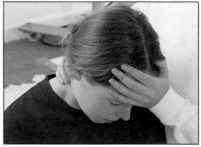

1. *Support the weight of the receiver's head as she relaxes it forward.*

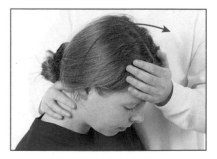

2. *Move her head slightly from side to side to give a stretch to the sides of her neck.*

I n half kneeling beside the receiver, using your leg to support her back, rest her forehead in your palm. Place your other hand on the back of her neck. Ask her to 'give her head' to your palm, allowing her head to come forward progressively as she relaxes more. This will give a mild 'opening stretch' to the back of her neck. Now move her head and neck slightly from side to side, giving a mild stretch to the sides of her neck. Slowly bring her head back up, emphasizing that she should remain totally relaxed and not contribute any movement herself.

NOTE THIS TECHNIQUE SHOULD BE DONE VERY SLOWLY TO AVOID THE RECEIVER TENSING UP. IF SHE HAS ANY NECK PROBLEM, AVOID THE TECHNIQUE UNTIL YOU ARE MORE FULLY TRAINED.

Child pose low back stretch

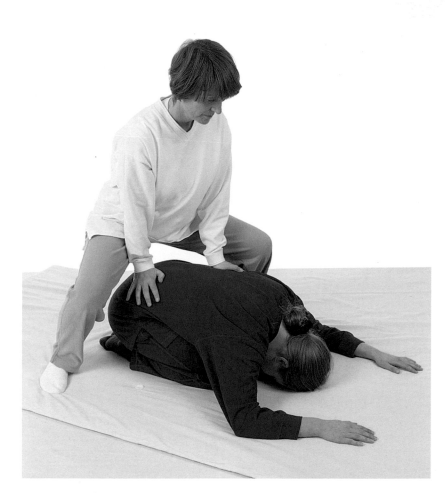

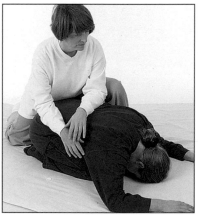

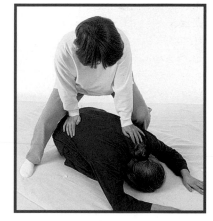

Have the receiver kneel with her head on the floor. If necessary she can raise her buttocks on a cushion. From standing or half kneeling, place one hand on one side of her lumbar area and the other hand on the opposite buttock. Apply a diagonal stretch. To develop your skill, try the movement using your forearms as well. Avoid leaning too high up her back because that will compress her neck and squash her face into the floor.

As an alternative to using your hands, try using your forearms.

Incorrect technique: if your hands are placed too high up the receiver's back, you will compress her neck and squash her face into the floor.

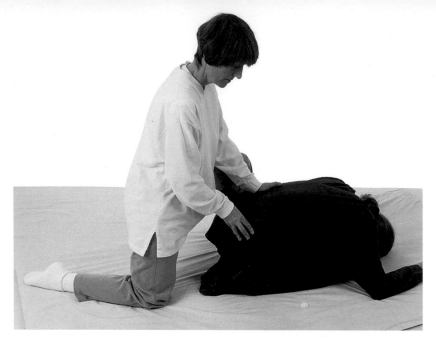

Back dispersal

This technique can be done with the receiver kneeling with her head on the floor or sitting or kneeling upright. Vigorously disperse tension and stiffness from the hip and buttock area with the heel of your hand or your fingertips. Alternatively, use hacking or cupping (see right), in which case you should avoid the kidney area. Repeat on the shoulder-blade area.

This type of 'back dispersal' technique is more common within other forms of Oriental bodywork. However, it is a good instant remedy for the receiver if she feels stiff around the hips, buttocks or shoulder-blades after a prolonged period of sitting.

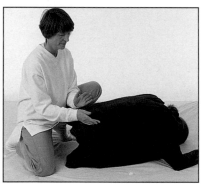

Hacking (chopping with the heel of your hand) on the buttock area.

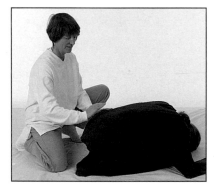

Cupping (slapping with hollowed palms) on the buttock area.

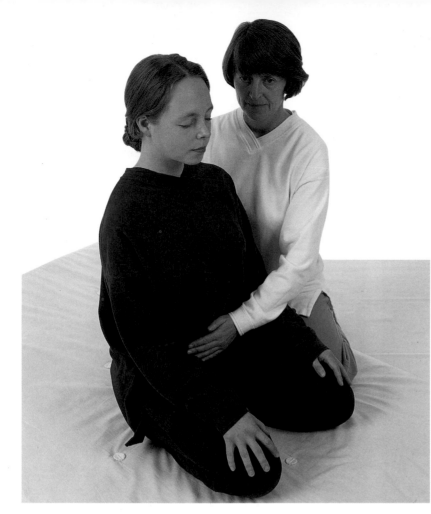

Hara/sacrum support

In this technique the receiver kneels or sits upright. Kneel beside her, facing her side. Hold her hara and sacrum simultaneously, tuning into her breathing rhythm.

This is a good way to finish the sitting sequence and indeed the foundation course sequence as a whole. Holding the hara and sacrum is very energizing for the receiver because you are helping her to become more aware of this area through making contact with her centre – the core of her body and the source of her vitality.

When you remove your hands very slowly to finish, the receiver will be so focused on her belly that she will experience a sensation akin to your hands being still in place. This indicates that her mind is now more attuned with the sensations of her body.

Appendix I

AN OVERVIEW
OF TRADITIONAL ORIENTAL BODYWORK

The blanket term for traditional Chinese bodywork is An Mo (Anma or Amma in Japanese). An Mo literally means 'press' (An) and 'rub' (Mo), which is a somewhat inadequate title because a wide variety of techniques and principles is involved. An Mo has four major branches, each one defined by the specialized techniques which characterize it. The four branches of An Mo are: General massage (Pu Tong An Mo); Push-Grab method (Tui Na An Mo); Cavity Press method (Dian Xue An Mo); and Ki method (Qi An Mo).

GENERAL MASSAGE
(Pu Tong An Mo or Anma)

Pu Tong An Mo is generally referred to simply as An Mo (or Anma in Japan). It requires no detailed knowledge of Ki channels or Oriental medicine theory. In both China and Japan, many of the practitioners are blind. This is because blind people cannot see the receiver's undressed body, so that in the older, more puritanical societies, there was less embarrassment when being massaged.

The core technique of Pu Tong An Mo is similar to the muscle-kneading technique practised by practitioners of Swedish massage. The aim of this form of massage is to relax body and mind, to allow Ki and blood to circulate smoothly, and to remove the aches and pains caused by an accumulation of waste products in the muscles after hard exercise. Mostly, however, it is used as a means of enjoyment.

PUSH-GRAB METHOD
(Tui Na An Mo)

Tui Na An Mo is usually just called Tui Na. It is named according to its two basic technique categories: Tui (push) and Na (grab to control). Tui Na has two distinct branches, one for treating injuries such as bruising and injuries to ligaments, tendons, joints and bones, the other for treating specific illnesses. Therefore, it requires a sound understanding of Oriental medicine principles.

Tui Na for injuries is commonly practised within the field of martial arts, where such injuries are common. In this context it is called 'fall strike method' (Die Da) to reflect its martial arts application. This type of Tui Na developed from an earlier system of bone and joint realignment.

Tui Na for illness is often used instead of acupuncture in situations where needling is difficult (such as with children, who tend to move and therefore bend or break the needles), or where the recipient is 'needle shy'. For this reason, it has been employed extensively in the treatment of young children since at least the beginning of the Ming dynasty.

Tui Na is becoming increasingly popular outside the Orient as a result of a more liberal attitude by the Chinese towards researching, reasserting and disseminating their heritage of traditional medicine.

CAVITY PRESS METHOD
(Dian Xue An Mo)

This method of bodywork focuses on stimulating acupressure points (tsubo in Japanese), Dian Xue literally meaning 'point cavity'. The pressure used in Dian Xue is more direct and penetrating than that used in Tui Na, which focuses more on the soft tissues. Therefore, Dian Xue can be viewed as the main precursor of Shiatsu, although aspects of Tui Na and particularly Qi An Mo (see below) also contributed. History suggests that it was first initiated by martial artists and later fully developed by physicians.

In China today, many Tui Na practitioners are also versed in Dian Xue, so it is not uncommon to find Point Cavity Push-Grab (Dian Xue Tui Na) practitioners.

KI METHOD
(Qi An Mo)

Ki method is the art of transferring or transmitting Ki from the giver to the receiver. It is also known as 'Curing with External Ki' (Wai Qi Liao Fa). Ki method is divided into two categories, one involving direct body contact and the other using no body contact. The body contact method is further sub-divided into a Ki projection method and a Ki resonance method. Ki projection method is used to supplement acupressure techniques (Dian Xue) insofar as the physician will project their own Ki into the acupressure point to nourish deficient Ki or remove excess Ki. Ki resonance method involves the practitioner lightly touching the receiver's skin to allow their Ki to correspond or 'resonate' with the receiver's Ki. Methods akin to these are currently being explored by many shiatsu practitioners in both the East and the West.

The non-contact Ki method is very similar to the Ki resonance method except that the practitioner does not actually make contact with the body, instead holding their fingertips or palm a few centimetres away from the receiver and directing Ki towards or away from specific areas of their body. It is what we would recognize today as Qigong healing.

Appendix II

THE APPLICATION OF YIN-YANG THEORY IN TCM

The following chart shows anatomy, physiology and pathology in the light of Yin and Yang. However, it must be remembered that Yin and Yang are relative to one another.

YIN	YANG
ANATOMY	
Lower part (body)	Upper part (head)
Interior (internal organs)	Exterior (skin, muscles)
Medial (Yin channels)	Lateral (Yang channels)
Front (Yin channels)	Back (Yang channels)
PHYSIOLOGY	
Store vital substances	Digest and excrete
Substance	Activity
Blood and body fluids	Ki
Down-bearing	Upward-moving
Inward movement	Outward movement
Yin moves energy	Yang moves energy
(and substances down to anus and urethra)	(and substances out to skin and limbs)
PATHOLOGY	
Cold (feelings of cold, aversion to cold, chills)	Hot (feelings of heat, aversion to heat, fever)
Quiet (sleepiness, aversion to movement/talking)	Restless (insomnia, tremors, fidgeting)
Wet (watery eyes, runny nose, loose stools, discharges)	Dry (eyes, nose, mouth, stools)
Soft (lumps and swellings	Hard (lumps and swellings)
Inhibition (hypoactivity)	Excitement (hyperactivity)
Slowness (movement, speech)	Rapidity (movement, speech)
Chronic disease	Acute disease
Gradual onset	Rapid onset
Lingering disease	Rapid changes
Likes to be covered	Throws off blankets
Pale face	Red face
Shallow breathing	Coarse breathing

CAUTION If someone has a red face this is a Yang symptom (because red is the most Yang colour), but it could be due either to a true excess of Yang or to deficiency of Yin (so that Yang is predominent relative to Yin). This doesn't distinguish between them. In Chinese medicine, pathology is seen as a pattern of disharmony. Commonly occurring patterns are called syndromes. In the syndrome Heart Fire (an excess pattern) it is common to have a red face, but you could also have a red face with Heart Yin Deficiency (a deficient pattern), or with Liver Fire or Liver Yin Deficiency, or indeed with a number of other syndromes. For the practitioner, the implications for treatment are: for an excess, treatment should be dispersing, for a deficiency, tonifying. So knowing that a red face is a Yang symptom is not sufficient information to reach a clear diagnosis and treatment principle. Yin and Yang are general categories which don't always give sufficient information to be useful clinically.

APPLICATION OF THE INTERACTIONS OF YIN-YANG

The interdependence of Yin-Yang is seen in the interactions between the organs: the Yin organs need the Yang ones to move substances about freely and clear out wastes, while the Yang ones need the Yin organs to nourish and restore them.

The inter-consuming of Yin-Yang: If you eat a large tub of ice cream (excess Yin) you are likely to suffer pain, bloating of the abdomen, cold limbs and aversion to cold, because the excessive Yin has consumed Yang, causing contraction, stagnation (pain) and cold.

The inter-transforming of Yin-Yang: Excessive work (Yang) without rest causes deficiency (Yin) of energy. Another example would be cold outside temperature invading the body causing chills, headache, runny nose (cold), eventually leading to fever and a cough with sticky yellow phlegm (heat).

The division of each organ's function into its Yin and its Yang aspects is an example of the application of the principle of divisibility of Yin and Yang. We talk of Kidney-Yin and Kidney-Yang, of Heart-Yin and Heart-Yang, of Liver-Yin and Liver-Yang. These terms are commonly used of the Yin organs rather than the Yang organs.

Appendix III

FIVE ELEMENT THEORY

The Five Elements interact in three main ways that are relevant to Oriental medicine. These are known as the Cosmological cycle, the Creation cycle and the Controlling cycle.

THE COSMOLOGICAL CYCLE

The first known reference to the Five Elements is the Cosmological cycle, in which the Elements were listed as water, fire, wood, metal and earth.

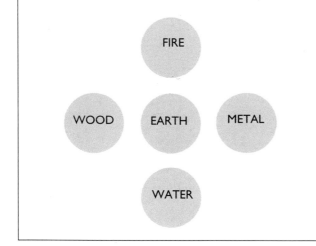

THE CREATION CYCLE

The diagram below represents the Creation cycle, also known as the Generating cycle or the Shen cycle. In the Creation cycle each Element creates or generates the one which succeeds it in the cycle and is in turn created by the one which precedes it. This is known as Mother–Child relationship between Elements. Each Element is the Mother of its succeeding Element and the Child of its preceding one.

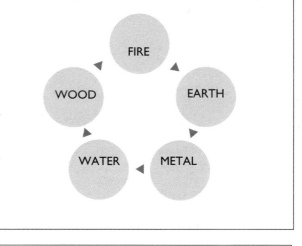

THE COSMOLOGICAL CYCLE

Water is the first-mentioned Element and is placed at the bottom: it is the basis of the sequence, the foundation of all the other elements. This concept is central to Oriental medical thinking: Water and specifically the Kidneys are the root of Yin and Yang, the foundation of all the other organs, the starting point of good health. Fire is placed opposite Water, at the top of the cycle. This reflects the fundamental opposition of Yin and Yang and the idea that Fire and Water oppose yet balance one another. There is direct communication between Water below and Fire above, as they are at the two extremities of a common axis. This idea translates in medical terms into the notion that Yin Water must flow upward to nourish the Heart, while the Fire of the Heart must flow downward to warm the Kidneys; also Essence must be strong (Kidneys and Water) for the Mind (Heart and Fire) to flourish.

In the centre, the middle, is Earth. The Stomach and Spleen play the principal role in nourishing all the organs,

THE CONTROLLING CYCLE

Also known as the Restraining cycle or the Ko cycle. In this cycle each Element controls or restrains the next but one in the cycle and is controlled by the last but one before it.

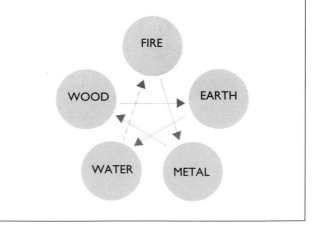

FIVE ELEMENT THEORY

Each Element or phase stands for many related qualities and correspondences. All phenomena can be classified according to the Five Elements: planets, animals, directions, seasons, sounds, odours, emotions.

THE MOST COMMONLY USED CORRESPONDENCES

	WOOD	FIRE	EARTH	METAL	WATER
Direction	East	South	Centre	West	North
Season	Spring	Summer	Late summer	Autumn	Winter
Climate	Wind	Heat	Dampness	Dryness	Cold
Process	Birth	Growth	Transforming	Harvest	Storage
Activity	Initiating	Peak	Balance	Decline	Rest
Time	Morning	Noon	Late afternoon	Evening	Night
Colour	Green	Red	Yellow	White	Blue/ black
Taste	Sour	Bitter	Sweet	Pungent	Salty
Smell	Rancid	Scorched	Fragrant	Rotten	Putrid
Zang	Liver	Heart/ Heart Protector	Spleen	Lung	Kidney
Fu	GB	Small Intestine/ Triple Heater	Stomach	Large Intestine	Bladder
Sense organ	Eyes	Tongue	Mouth	Nose	Ears
Tissue	Tendons/ ligaments	Blood vessels	Flesh	Skin/ body hair	Bones
Body Fluid	Tears	Sweat	Saliva	Mucus	Urine
Emotion	Anger	Joy	Worry	Grief	Fear
Sound	Shouting	Laughter	Singing	Weeping	Groaning
Mind	Planning/ controlling	Love/ sensitivity	Concentration/ analysing	Taking in/ letting go	Endurance/ will
Spiritual	Ethereal soul/ Hun	Consciousness/ Shen	Intellect/ Yi	Corporeal soul/ Po	Willpower/ Zhi
Energetic directions	Ascending and dispersing	Radiating in all directions	Centre, up and down	Descending and dispersing	Floating or suspended

because they digest food and provide Ki for the body. The Heart especially relies on them to provide Ki for the production and pumping of Blood. So the Stomach and Spleen are considered to be the main source of Ki and Blood produced after birth from food and air, called the Post-Heaven Ki. Therefore, whenever there is deficiency of Ki and Blood in the body it may be useful to tonify and strengthen the Earth Element in order to provide Ki and Blood for other organs.

Finally this arrangement of Fire, Earth and Water reflects the idea of heaven above, earth below and human beings in the centre which is central to the Oriental view of the universe. Wood is placed on the left and its energy ascends and goes outwards and Metal is placed on the right, its energy descending and spreading or dispersing.

THE CREATION CYCLE

Wood burns so it is said to be the Mother of Fire. It is also the child of Water. Fire creates ashes so it is said to be the Mother of Earth; it is also the Child of Wood. Earth contains metal ores: it is said to be the Mother of Metal; it is also the Child of Fire. Metal melts (becomes liquid): it is said to be the Mother of Water; it is also the Child of Earth. Water nourishes Wood so it is the Mother of Wood; it is also the Child of Metal.

THE CONTROLLING CYCLE

Wood penetrates Earth so Wood is said to control Earth (plant roots binding soil together). Earth channels Water and is said to control it (rivers and lakes are contained by their surrounding earth banks). Water extinguishes Fire: Water is said to control Fire. Fire melts Metal: Fire is said to control Metal. Metal cuts Wood: Metal is said to control Wood.

If any element is excessive or deficient, this will in turn affect other Elements along one or the other, or indeed both, cycles. If the effect of imbalance is felt along the creation cycle then either the Mother or the Child Element is affected; this can be either the Mother affecting the Child or conversely the Child affecting the Mother. The Mother can affect the Child by not nourishing it enough. The Child can affect the Mother by drawing too much from her and weakening her.

If the effect of imbalance is felt along the controlling cycle it can result in overacting, or over-controlling of one Element by another. This follows the normal cycle, but is simply an excess of controlling. Fire normally controls Metal, but if Fire is excessive it can act too powerfully upon Metal and damage it. This is overacting, also sometimes called invading.

Counteracting or rebelling is the other effect that can occur along the controlling cycle. This occurs when the controlling cycle goes into reverse at some point – for example Fire controls Metal but if Fire is weak and Metal is strong then Metal can attack Fire instead of being controlled by it. This is counteracting or rebelling, sometimes called 'insulting'. If an element is in excess it will tend to overact on the element it usually controls and it will also tend to rebel against the element that usually controls it.

Practical application

In terms of the practical application of Five Element theory many of the correspondences are useful clinically. Taking Wood and the Liver as an example: people with Liver imbalances (in the Oriental medicine sense of Ki imbalance, rather than the Western physiological sense) will often have a greenish tinge to their complexion, their voice may also be quite loud, they may be irritable and feel worse for windy weather.

The eyes relate to the Liver but it is not the only organ that can affect the eyes. The Heart Channel has an internal branch which goes to the eyes, the Gall Bladder and Triple Heater channels begin and end respectively near them, and indeed problems unrelated to internal organ pathology may affect them. In other words, though Five Element theory says that the eyes relate to the Liver, clinically the facts are more complicated. The model has its limitations and it is therefore unwise to rely on the Five Element model of correspondences alone for diagnosis.

The cosmological, creation and controlling cycles provide a model of a dynamic balance between the elements. If the balance is upset, disease ensues. If the cosmological cycle is affected and if the Kidneys (Water) are weak, this will directly affect both the Spleen (Earth) and the Heart (Fire), causing weakness in one or both. In the case of the creation cycle, if the Kidneys are weak, this will impact on the Liver (Wood), causing deficiency. In the case of the controlling cycle, if the Ki of the Liver stagnates it may overact on the Spleen, disrupting digestion. This is called Liver invading the Spleen and it is a commonly seen pattern. Lungs overacting on Liver, however, is not a common pattern. In other words the model may be a useful tool to interpret some clinical facts, but should not be applied too rigidly.

For the shiatsu therapist, the Five Element model is useful insofar as it can help them understand the reason behind their diagnosis. In some situations, it can also influence their treatment strategy.

Appendix IV

METAPHORS TO EXPLAIN KYO-JITSU

Your approach to a kyo or jitsu tsubo can be equated with the way you might approach a herd of deer grazing in a meadow. In a small clearing in the woods to one side of the meadow, two stags are locked in conflict over who is to be the dominant male of the herd. This situation arises during the mating season, but on this occasion the stag conflict is heightened by the fact that a fawn has been badly injured. The stags' innate desire to become the dominant male sire is exacerbated by an instinct to be the chief protector of the herd.

TONIFYING 'BLOCKED/FULL' JITSU (doomed to failure)

Imagine that these deer are relatively tame, so you could get close to them if you approached with care. You want to come close to the stags to study their aggressive behaviour, but that would not be a good idea because the stags are confined within the clearing in the woods and very much preoccupied with their struggle. There is already too much tense energy around and your presence would add to it. If you persist in trying to get between them, the aggression of both stags will increase and they will turn on you. They do not want you around any more than a jitsu tsubo would want your thumb trying to get into it. The sensible thing is to leave the stags alone for now.

DISPERSING 'BLOCKED/FULL' JITSU (without tonifying kyo)

If you collected some friends together and rushed at the stags, making as much noise and commotion as possible, they would scatter, at which point you and your friends would leave the scene. For a while, the concentrated activity in that corner of the woods has been forcibly removed.

However, when the coast is clear the stags return to this favoured place of conflict. If you and your friends rushed them again the stags may not scatter so easily a second time, being more accustomed to your presence. This is akin to dispersing jitsu by applying active technique directly to it, but without directing it to a kyo area. The Ki scatters randomly, only to return to the same place later on with more tenacity and stubbornness.

CALMING 'HYPERACTIVE' JITSU

Standing on the edge of the scene is a young stag who is becoming excited. Though he is rather slight in build and but a shadow of the hefty mature stags, he is frenetically rushing around, filling his space with jittery energy. You approach him and offer him a handful of grass, which he finds quite appealing. You then radiate a very serene demeanour, holding your calming hand to his back. The young stag eventually settles down to graze calmly, because deep down he knows that he is not sufficiently mature to engage in mating rituals. This is like placing a calming hand on the type of jitsu which does not represent excess quantity of Ki, but rather excess activity within a limited quantity of Ki.

TONIFYING MILD RATHER THAN CHRONIC KYO, THAT IS, RESISTANCE AT THE SURFACE (simultaneously dispersing jitsu via two-hand connection)

The wounded fawn's mother and a few other relatives are staying close to the fawn to protect it. You are there with a first aid kit, intending to help the fawn. But how are those protecting the fawn to know you want to help? To them you pose a threat, but they also have a sixth sense suggesting that you might in fact be trying to help. They are confused, so you approach very slowly, stopping whenever there is a hint of panic. You give enough space and time for them to become accustomed to the idea of your offer to help. At no stage must you assume acceptance and rush in to finish the job. The same can apply to a kyo tsubo. Sometimes you detect a 'need' for more Ki, but when you try to apply perpendicular pressure, surrounding Ki aggregates at the neck of the tsubo, preventing further entry.

Once you reach the fawn and you are clearly helping it rather than harming it, its protectors back off a little and the whole scene becomes more relaxed. You administer some medicine which gives the fawn some vitality (some Ki) and it struggles to its feet.

COMPARATIVE RESPONSE OF BLOCKED, HYPERACTIVE OR EMPTY 'NEEDY' TSUBO TO STATIONARY PERPENDICULAR PRESSURE

The longer you stay motionless at the mouth of the kyo tsubo the more the resistance dissipates, allowing you further entry as long as you do not push. Conversely, the longer you linger at the mouth of the full jitsu tsubo, the more intolerant the Ki becomes and resistance actually increases. The only way to deal with the jitsu which is more frenetic than full is to use a palm rather than a thumb; to be calm and allow that calmness to subdue the jitsu activity. This is very similar in attitude to dealing with the protected kyo tsubo, except you would not try to enter the tsubo to add Ki.

TONIFYING MORE CHRONIC, BUT NOT THE MOST CHRONIC, KYO (flaccid kyo)

Another scenario could be this: the fawn is completely unconscious and inert. The herd have left it for dead and are grazing several hundred metres away. However, the mother remains on the edge of the herd, keeping the fawn in sight. You can approach the fawn with no resistance. When you reach it, you patiently administer some healing factor (Ki). After a while, the fawn stirs. This is noticed by the mother, who comes over to the fawn, along with others of the herd. You leave and allow the herd to support the revived fawn.

TONIFYING VERY CHRONIC KYO (stiff kyo)

Yet another scenario: the fawn is dead and the herd is on the horizon. Even the mother deer has given up hope and forgotten about the fawn. You approach the fawn to see how it is. There is no resistance to your approach, but what you find when you reach the fawn is a stiff, inert carcass, analogous to a stiff, inert kyo tsubo.

When something is dead, the Ki, blood and body fluids no longer circulate to moisten, activate and nourish the body. When the creature has been dead for a while, the prolonged absence of Ki, blood and fluid function will result in a general drying and stiffening of the tissues. Likewise, kyo in part of a living body reflects the relative lack of life (Ki) in that part of the body. If the Ki is very deficient for a long time, blood and fluid circulation to that area will be drastically reduced, causing a drying out and atrophy of the tissues. The chronic kyo area will be virtually a 'dead' part of the body; a part that the owner will have very little awareness of, unless it is so dead that the tissues exhibit pathological problems (an extreme example would be gangrene).

No matter how much healing agent you give the fawn, it is dead and that is that. No matter how long you try to tonify that completely stiff, dead kyo, it will not respond. So what can you do? It makes more sense if, rather than concentrating on the dead fawn itself, you think of it in terms of the space it is occupying being a dead space. All around, active creatures are bringing their living space alive.

Because you persist in standing over the carcass, you mark the spot and eventually attract the attention of various predators, carrion feeders and other opportunists. In due course, the predators will come closer, and when you move off they will eat the carcass, effectively causing renewed activity in that space and thereby bringing life to it.

Translated into the chronic stiff kyo situation, this means that if you hold patient, sustained perpendicular pressure on that lifeless tsubo, nothing whatsoever will happen. However, if you leave it and tonify and disperse more interactive parts of the body you might well find that when you return, either during this treatment or within a later treatment, some activity has begun to manifest in that formerly stiff kyo tsubo.

Appendix V

THE CHINESE CHANNEL CLOCK CYCLE

The 12 primary channels are all linked together in one
continuous loop, so if you could pull them out, unravel them
and lay them on the ground you would get a huge unbroken
circle. Ki flows continuously around the loop, peaking in each
channel in turn for a two-hour period. This causes each channel
to be particularly active for the same period each day. This does
not mean the channel is necessarily more jitsu during that time;
this is more akin to an underlying wave of Ki. Having said
that, a chronically jitsu channel will tend to be more blocked
or hyperactive with Ki during its 'peak' time.

THE CHANNEL CLOCK CYCLE

	Ki 'peaking' in channel	Ki 'low point' in channel
3.00am – 5.00am	Lungs	Bladder
5.00am – 7.00am	Large Intestine	Kidneys
7.00am – 9.00am	Stomach	Heart Protector
9.00am – 11.00am	Spleen	Triple Heater
11.00am – 1.00pm	Heart	Gall Bladder
1.00pm – 3.00pm	Small Intestine	Liver
3.00pm – 5.00pm	Bladder	Lungs
5.00pm – 7.00pm	Kidneys	Large Intestine
7.00pm – 9.00pm	Heart Protector	Stomach
9.00pm – 11.00pm	Triple Heater	Spleen
11.00pm – 1.00am	Gall Bladder	Heart
1.00am – 3.00am	Liver	Small Intestine

Doing shiatsu or Makko-ho exercises on or to a channel during its Ki peak is most effective, although not particularly convenient if the peak happens to be from 3.00am to 5.00am. However, it is also effective to address the channel when it is furthest from its Ki peak, which is 12 hours later. Therefore, if the Lung channel peaks between 3.00am and 5.00am, it is useful to do a Lung Makko-ho exercise between 3.00pm and 5.00pm.

Appendix VI

CHANNEL DIAGRAMS

The channels, also known as Meridians, are the pathways through the body along which Ki flows. There are 12 major channels, each linked to the function of a particular organ, plus two extra channels that run up the midline of the torso and head on the front and back. The channel pathways run in a circuitous route through and around the body. They rise at intervals on to the surface, to give us the surface pathways as depicted in this appendix, and dip deeper into the body to connect with the internal organs.

In the same way that arteries sub-divide into arterioles, which in turn sub-divide into capillaries, the major or 'classical' channels have extensions to their distribution and wider connections with other minor channels to create a network over and throughout the body. In fact, all parts of the body are touched by Ki brought to them by the channels via their sub-divisions and branches. The detailed location of minor channels and channel extensions are not relevant to the contents of this book and are thus not shown.

Each major channel is paired with another channel. In general, the channels which exist more on the front of the body are Yin channels, as they relate to Yin organs and because the front of the body is more Yin than the back (see Yin-Yang theory, pages 10–12). Conversely, the channels which exist on the back of the body are Yang channels as they relate to Yang organs and because the back of the body is more Yang than the front.

There are 12 channels that mirror themselves bilaterally on the body, meaning that the channel map for the left half of the body is a mirror image of the right side of the body. The Conception Vessel and Governing Vessel are single pathways because they circulate the midline of the head and torso.

NOTE: The location of tsubos along the channels are frequently measured in multiples of 'cun'. A 'cun' is a unit of measurement used in oriental medicine which is approximately equivalent to the recipient's thumb at its widest part.

Lung

1 1 cun below 2 in the 1st intercostal space, 6 cun lateral to the anterior midline.

2 In the depression of the infraclavicular fossa, 6 cun lateral to the anterior midline, level with the lower border of the sternal extremity of the clavicle.

5 In the transverse cubital crease in the depression on the radial side of the tendon of biceps brachii muscle.

7 On the radial side of the forearm, proximal to the styloid process of the radius, 1.5 cun proximal to the wrist crease.

9 At the radial end of the wrist crease, where the radial artery is palpable.

11 On the radial side of the thumb, 0.1 cun proximal to the corner of the nail.

Large Intenstine

1 On the radial side of the index finger, 0.1 cun proximal to the corner of the nail.

4 Between the 1st and 2nd matacarpal bones on the radial side of the midpoint of the 2nd metacarpal bone.

5 On the radial end of the wrist crease in the depression between the tendons of short extensor and long extensor muscles of the thumb, when the thumb is tilted upwards.

10 On the radial side of the dorsal surface of the forearm on the line connecting 5 and 11, 2 cun below the cubital crease.

11 At the lateral end of the cubital crease when the elbow is flexed.

15 In the depression anterior and inferior to the acromion when the arm is abducted.

16 On the shoulder in the depression between the acromial extremity of the clavicle and the spine of the scapula.

18 Between the two heads of the sternocleidomastoid muscle at the level of the laryngeal protuberance.

20 In the nasolabial groove at the level of the midpoint of the lateral border of the nasal ala.

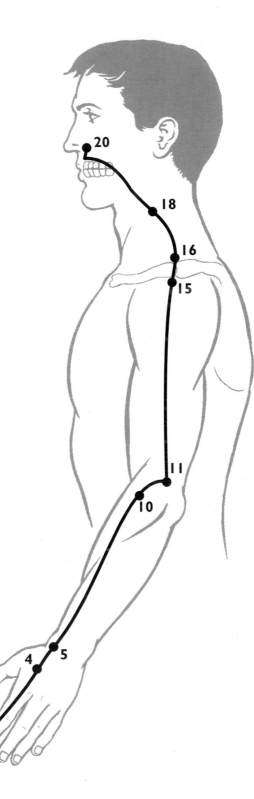

Stomach

1 Directly below the pupil (when looking straight ahead) on the inferior ridge of the orbital cavity.

3 Directly inferior to 1 on the inferior border of ala nasi.

9 At the level of the laryngeal prominence on the anterior border of the sternocleidomastoid where the pulse of cartoid artery can be felt.

18 4 cun lateral to the midline in the 5th intercostal space directly inferior to the nipple.

25 2 cun lateral to the midline at the level of the umbilicus.

34 2 cun superior to the lateral superior border of the patella.

36 In th depression 3 cun inferior to 35 (in the lateral eye of the knee) and 1 cun lateral to the crest of the tibia.

40 Midway between the level of the lateral malleolus and 35 and 2 cun lateral to the crest of the tibia.

41 At the level of the tip of the lateral malleolus on the anterior aspect of the ankle between the tendons of extensor digitorum longus and hallucis longus muscles.

42 1.3 cun distal to 41 at the high point of the dorsum of the foot in the depression formed by the 2nd and 3rd metatarsal bones and the cunieform bone, where the pulse of the dorsal artery can be felt.

44 In the web of the 2nd and 3rd toes in the depression distal and lateral to the 2nd matatarsophalangeal joint.

45 0.1 cun proximal to the lateral corner of the base of the 2nd toenail.

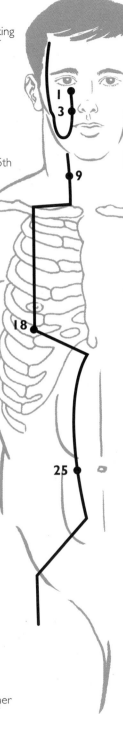
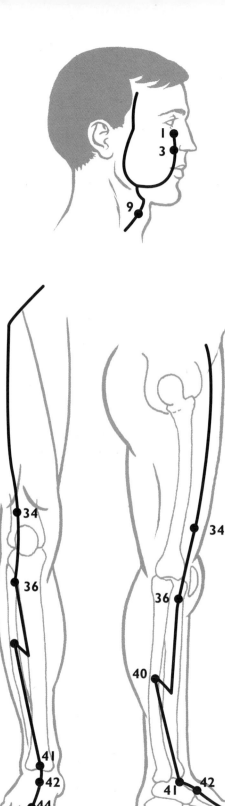

Spleen

1 0.1 cun below the medial corner of the base of the big toenail.

3 Proximal and inferior to the head of the 1st metatarsal bone on the junction of the dark and light skin.

6 3 cun superior to the vertex of the medial malleolus on the posterior border of the tibia.

9 On the inferior border of the medial condyle of the tibia in the depression on the posterior border of the tibia.

10 2 cun above the superior medial border of the patella on the medial margin of the vastus medialis muscle.

15 4 cun lateral to the midline at the level of the umbilicus.

21 In the 6th inter-costal space, 6 cun below the centre of the axilla.

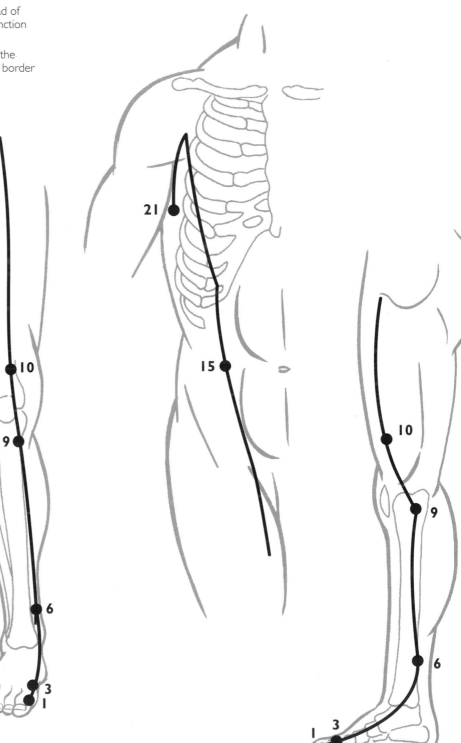

Heart

1 At the apex of the axillary fossa, where the pulsation of the axillary artery is possible.

3 With the elbow flexed, at the midpoint of the line connecting the medial end of the cubital crease and the medial epicondyle of the humerus.

7 At the ulnar end of the wrist crease in the depression on the radial side of the tendon of ulnar flexor muscle.

9 On the radial side of the little finger, 0.1 cun proximal to the corner of the nail.

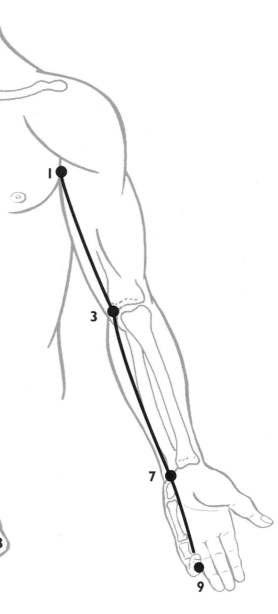

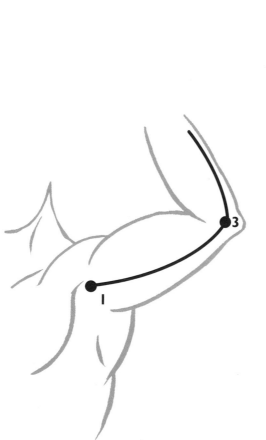

Small Intestine

1 On the ulnar side of the little finger, 0.1 cun proximal to the corner of the nail.

3 At the ulnar end of the distal palmar crease, on the junction of the pale and dark skin, proximal to the 5th metacarpophalangeal joint when the hollow fist is made.

4 In the depression between the proximal end of the 5th matacarpal bone and hamate bone on the junction of the pale and dark skin.

8 In the depression between the olecranon of the ulna and the medial epicondyle of the humerus.

10 Above the end of the posterior axillary fold, in the depression below the lower border of the spine of the scapula.

11 In the depression of the centre of the subscapula fossa inferior to the midpoint of the lower border of the spine of the scapula, at the level of the 4th thoracic vertebra.

17 Level with the angle of the mandible, on the anterior border of the sternocleidomastoid muscle.

18 Directly below the outer canthus of the eye in the depression on the lower border of the zygomatic bone.

19 Anterior to the tragus, where a depression is formed when the mouth is opened.

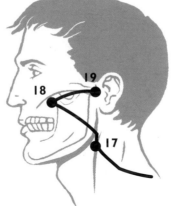

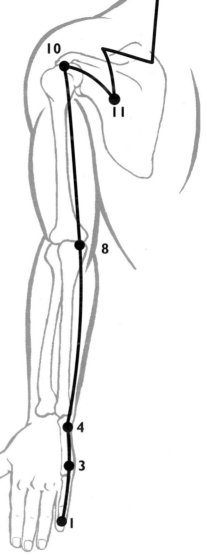

Bladder

1 In the depression slightly above the inner canthus of the eye.

2 In the depression at the medial end of the eyebrow in the supraorbital notch.

10 On the nape of the neck, in the depression of the lateral border of the trapezius muscle, 1.3 cun lateral to the midpoint of the posterior hairline.

13 Below the spinious process of the 3rd thoracic vertebra, 1.5 cun lateral to the posterior midline.

14 Below the spineous process of the 4th thoracic vertebra, 1.5 cun lateral to the posterior midline.

15 Below the spineous process of the 5th thoracic vertebra, 1.5 cun lateral to the posterior midline.

18 Below the spineous process of the 9th thoracic vertebra, 1.5 cun lateral to the posterior midline.

19 Below the spineous process of the 10th thoracic vertebra, 1.5 cun lateral to the posterior midline.

20 Below the spineous process of the 11th thoracic vertebra, 1.5 cun lateral to the posterior midline.

21 Below the spineous process of the 12th thoracic vertebra, 1.5 cun lateral to the posterior midline

22 Below the spineous process of the 1st lumbar vertebra, 1.5 cun lateral to the posterior midline.

23 Below the spineous process of the 2nd lumbar vertebra, 1.5 cun lateral to the posterior midline.

25 Below the spineous process of the 4th lumbar vertebra, 1.5 cun lateral to the posterior midline.

27 On the sacrum at the level of the 1st posterior sacral foramen, 1.5 cun lateral to the posterior midline.

28 On the sacrum at the level of the 2nd posterior sacral foramen, 1.5 cun lateral to the posterior midline.

40 At the midpoint of the popliteal crease between the tendons of muscle biceps femoris and semitendinosus.

57 Inferior to the belly of the gastrocnemius muscle between 40 and 60, in the depression formed when the heel is lifted.

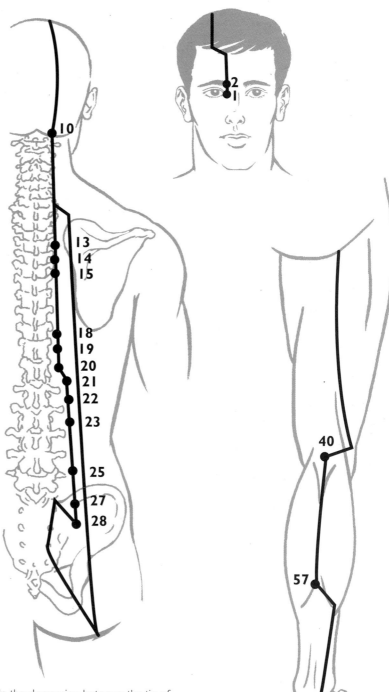

60 In the depression between the tip of the lateral malleolus and the Achilles tendon.

67 0.1 cun proximal to the lateral corner of the 5th toenail.

Kidney

1 In the depression on the anterior part of the sole when the foot is plantarflexed, approximately on the junction of the anterior third and posterior two thirds of the line connecting the base of the 2nd and 3rd toes and the heel.

3 In the depression between the tip of the medial malleolus and the Achilles tendon.

6 In the depression below the tip of the medial malleolus.

7 2 cun superior to 3 anterior to the Achilles tendon.

10 On the medial side of the popliteal fossa between the tendons of muscles semimembranosus and semitendinosus when the knee is flexed.

27 Inferior to the lower border of the clavicle 2 cun lateral to the midline.

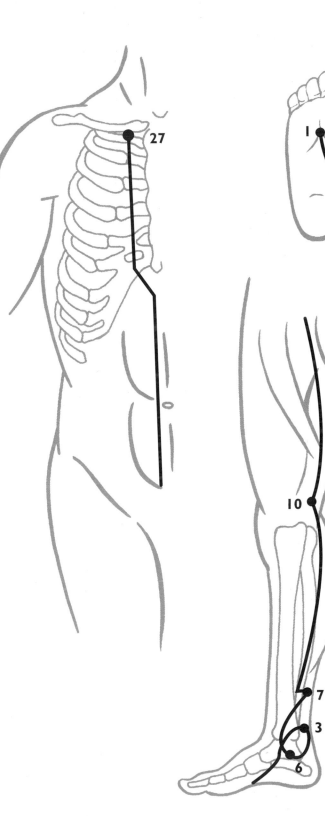

Heart Protector

1 1 cun lateral to the nipple in the 4th intercostal space.

3 On the transverse cubital crease on the ulnar side of the tendon of biceps brachii muscle.

6 2 cun proximal to the transverse crease of the wrist between the tendons on the pulmaris longus and flexor carpi radialis muscles.

7 On the wrist crease in the depression between the tendons of the palmaris longus and flexor carpi radialis muscles.

8 In the palm of the hand on the radial side of the 3rd metacarpal bone, proximal to the metacarpophalangeal joint.

9 In the middle of the tip of the 3rd finger.

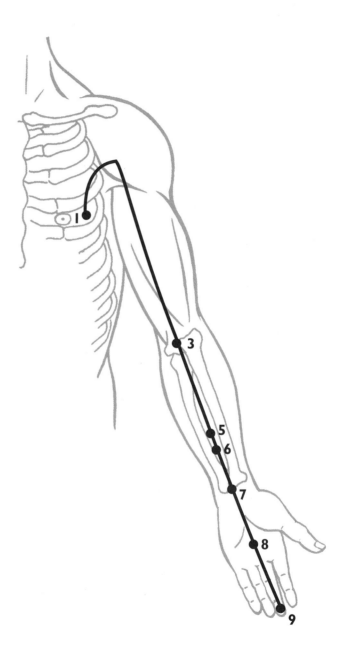

Triple Heater

1 0.1 cun proximal to the corner of the fourth fingernail on the ulnar side.

4 On the dorsum of the wrist in the depression lateral to tendon of extensor digitorum muscle.

5 2 cun proximal to 4, between the ulnar and radius.

10 1 cun above the olecranon in the depression formd when the elbow is flexed.

14 In the posterior depression below the ridge of the acromium when the arm is abducted.

17 Posterior to the earlobe between the tip of the mastoid process and the angle of the mandible.

23 In the depression at the lateral end of the eyebrow.

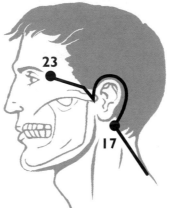

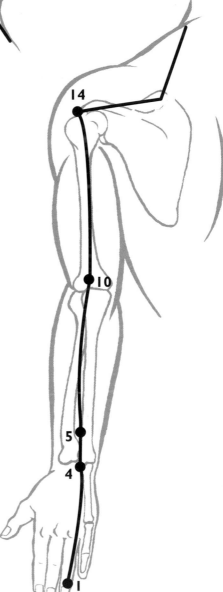

Gall Bladder

1 0.5 cun lateral to the outer canthus of the eye in the depression on the lateral border of the orbit.

12 In the depression inferior and posterior to the mastoid process.

20 Below the occipital bone, level with Governing Vessel 16, in the depression between the trapezius and sternocleido-mastoid muscles.

21 On the highest point of the shoulder, directly above the nipple, at the midpoint between Governing Vessel 14 and the acromion process.

24 On the mammilary line, 4 cun lateral to the midline, in the 7th intercostal space.

25 Below the free end of the 12th rib.

30 On the lateral side of the thigh, one third of the way between the greater trochanter of the femur and the sacral hiatus when the hip is flexed.

34 In the depression anterior and inferior to the head of the fibula.

40 Anterior and inferior to the lateral malleolus in the depression on the lateral side of the tendon of the extensor digitorum longus muscle.

44 0.1 cun proximal to the lateral corner of the fourth toenail.

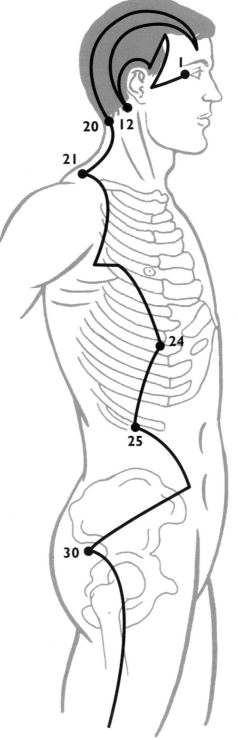

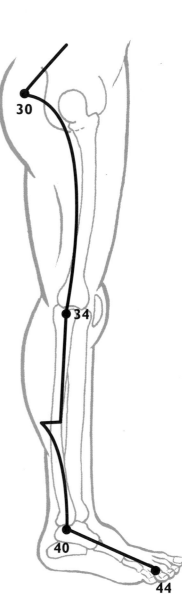

Liver

1 0.1 cun proximal to the lateral corner of the base of the big toenail.

3 On the dorsum of the foot, in the depression distal to the junction of the first and second metatarsal bones.

4 In the depression medial to the tendon of tibialis anterior, level with the tip of the medial malleolus.

8 On the medial side of the knee in the depression on the medial end of transverse popliteal crease between the upper border of the medial epicondyle of the femur and the tendon of muscle semimembranosus.

13 Below the free end of the 11th rib.

14 On the mamillary line, 4 cun lateral to the midline, in the 6th intercostal space.

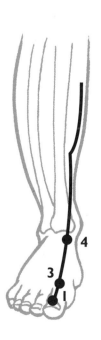

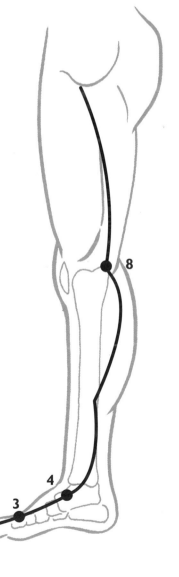

Conception Vessel

1 In the centre of the perineum.

3 On the anterior midline, 4 cun below the centre of the umbilicus.

4 On the anterior midline, 3 cun below the centre of the umbilicus.

5 On the anterior midline, 2 cun below the centre of the umbilicus.

6 On the anterior midline, 1.5 cun below the centre of the umbilicus.

8 At the centre of the umbilicus.

12 On the anterior midline, 4 cun above the centre of the umbilicus.

14 On the anterior midline, 6 cun above the centre of the umbilicus.

17 On the anterior midline, at the level of the 4th intercostal space, at the midpoint of the line connecting the nipples.

22 At the centre of the suprasternal fossa.

24 In the depression under the lower lip (at the midpoint of the mentolabial sulcus).

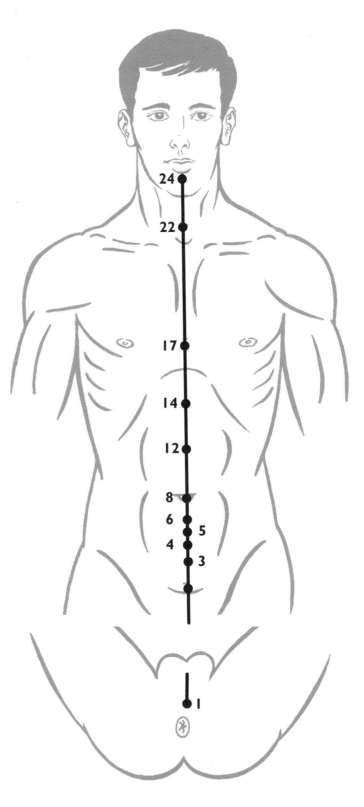

Governing Vessel

1 At the midpoint of the line connecting the tip of the coccyx and the anus.

4 On the posterior midline, in the depression below the spineous processes of the 2nd lumbar vertebra.

14 On the posterior midline, in the depression below the spineous process of the 7th cervical vertebra.

20 At the midpoint of the line connecting the apexes of both ears.

28 Inside the upper lip at the junction of the labial frenulum and the upper gum.

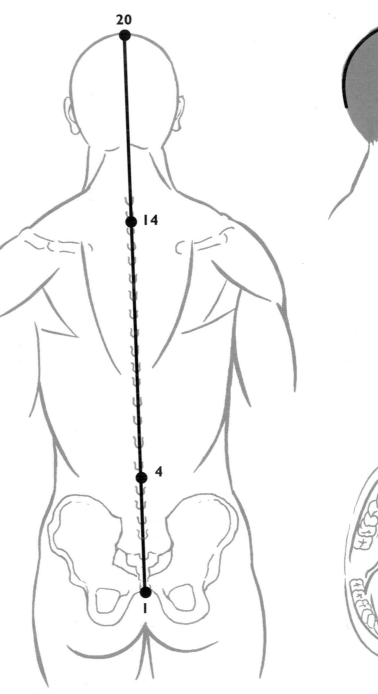

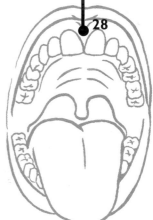

Index